The Belly Handbook

Eliminate that unwanted *Belly Fat* and KEEP IT OFF!

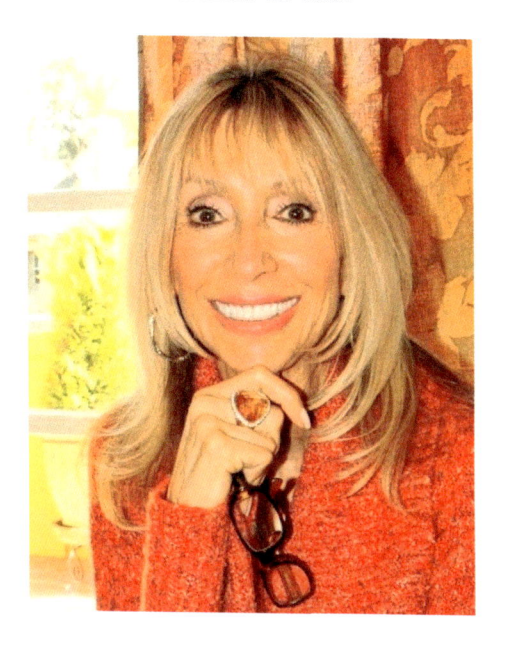

Barbara A. Hoffman

Your guide to a flatter stomach.
That day is here!

Rediscover your waist line with this **hormone balancing** plan

The Belly Flat Handbook

By Barbara A. Hoffman

Disclaimer:
This book is intended as a reference volume only, not as a medical manual. The information given here is designed to help you make informed decisions about your health.

The Belly Flat Handbook Copyright © 2018 by Barbara A. Hoffman. All rights reserved.

First Edition: February 2018. Printed in the USA.
ISBN: 978-0-9753353-3-8

Cover photo: Tony Florez Photography, Corona del Mar California

Trademarks
All terms mentioned in this book that are known to be trademarks or service marks have been appropriately capitalized. Trademarks belong to the appropriate companies.

About The Author

Barbara A. Hoffman

Barbara Hoffman is a Naturopath, medical researcher & journalist, women's health advocate and natural hormone and weight consultant.

For 13 years she produced a cable network television program which focused on health and wellness. Her continual studies and education and passion for women's health fuels her mission to empower women to seize control of their health. She will tirelessly encourage you in your goal to be the YOU that you want to be.

Barbara has been in the medical field for over 30 years and worked in the field of women's health since 1980. For all of those years she has been researching weight loss, the benefits of natural hormones over synthetic hormones, and the 35 symptoms of hormone imbalance, especially focusing on insomnia, hair loss, depression, anxiety and weight gain.

Barbara has a passion for women and men who are lugging around 20-40 unwanted extra pounds right around their mid-section. This plan can decrease and eliminate the infamous "Belly Fat"

Barbara resides in Orange County, California. She has been married for 35 years and has one son. She will often say that she considers people like you her "extended family" You can always email Barbara here: barbara@askbarbarahoffman.com She promises to answer!

Dedication

I lovingly thank all of you amazing women and men over the miles who have called, written and emailed over the years. Usually you pick up a book, read the dedication, and once again the author has dedicated a book to someone else and not to you. Not this time…this book is for you. Whether we have communicated or not, I trust that someday we will cross paths in some way and share a story, a smile, or a victory.

I promise to continue educating and encouraging you in your quest for Better Health Naturally. You are the reason I study and write because you are MY encouragement. You cannot truly appreciate how much I love to hear from you and to help you. I'll never stop advocating for you.

I extend my heartfelt thank you to the Daystar Television Network for promoting the message of hormone balance to God's people all around the world. Daystar is an abiding source of spiritual guidance. When I am tired or discouraged, God's word helps me to sing a new song every day. Thank you, Joni and Marcus and the Daystar family.

I am extraordinarily fortunate to have a beloved, youthful staff who keep me inspired on a daily basis…Kim, Aaron, Paula, Hilda, and Hannah. I am grateful for your beautiful hearts, laughter and joy and your dedication to every single person who calls or writes.

And the fact that you treat me like I am a youngster. Which I am NOT, but thank you for the subterfuge. Hugs and kisses all around.

To David, my delightfully delicious husband and my son, the writer and filmmaker, Drew. You keep me committed to teaching and working diligently all the time because I see your belief in me. Your quiet, powerful support needs to be shouted from the rooftops

I am so grateful to God. Long ago, I thought I had lost my way. I wanted to be a teacher or a writer and somehow I got "derailed" in my 20's. Then…
God put me on this glorious path. And now, I get to write, teach and rejoice in the new friends I have found along the way….YOU!

Thank you all SO much…and….Belly Fat Be Gone. I'm on your side and I won't give up on you.

With Love,

Your Friend,
Barbara Hoffman

"For we aim at what is honorable not only in the Lord's sight, but in the sight of man."
2 Corinthians 8:21

Table of Contents

Chapter 1:   Overview: A discussion of Hormone Imbalance regarding chapters 2-10……………….. 1

Chapter 2:   **Estrogen Dominance**………………..… 11

Chapter 3:   **Insulin Resistance**………….…............ 15

Chapter 4:   **High Insulin Recap**………………..…. 21

Chapter 5:   **High Cortisol**…………………………. 23

Chapter 6:   **Low Progesterone**…………………... 29

Chapter 7:   **Low DHEA**…………………………..… 33

Chapter 8:   **Low Melatonin**………………………… 35

Chapter 9:   **Low Thyroid**……………………….…. 39

Chapter 10: **Low Testosterone**……….......………. 43

Chapter 11: **Estrogen Detox**………………………. 45

Chapter 12: **Boost Your Fat Burners**…................ 53

Chapter 13: **Belly Fat and the Brain**…..…………. 59

Chapter 14: **Banish Cravings**……………………... 69

Chapter 15: **Beat the Bloat**………..…………..…. 73

Chapter 16: **Exercise and Belly Fat**……................ 77

Chapter 17: **Estrogen Dominance FAQ's** ………. 81

Chapter 18: **Belly Flat Supplements** ……..……. 85

Chapter 19: **6 Part Sugar Detox** ..…….………. 89

Chapter 20: **Final Thoughts**………………...…. 121

Chapter 1
Overview

"Help! Where did this Belly Fat come from? I'm not eating any differently! I look down and see a Pooch! No matter what I do as far as exercise or diet, I can't budge this unwanted fat"

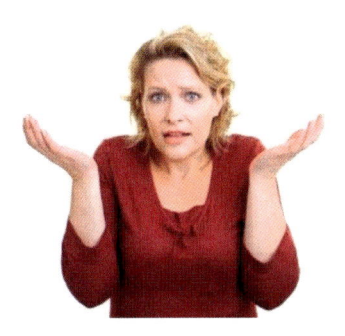

Have you gained unwanted weight around your waist and belly? Does it feel like it happened overnight? Are you tired of looking down and seeing the muffin top spill over your waistband? Are you discouraged, disheartened, embarrassed? Have you tried severe diets that did nothing for the belly fat? It's your hormones.

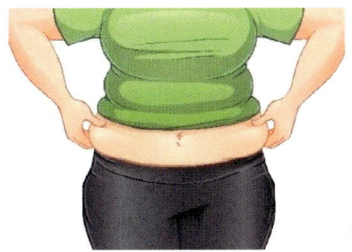

"Oh, no…Muffin Top!"

So many women call or write to me saying "I'm bloated" OR "I've got a pooch that I never had before" "The older I get, the bigger my belly gets. I diet and exercise and it never goes away" OR "my waist band is tight" OR "I suddenly have gained 20 pounds, it feels like it was almost overnight" OR "I feel like I swallowed a bowling ball" "I don't know what has gone wrong"

Maybe you are saying all of these. You are now desperate because you've been dieting, dieting, dieting, and the belly fat just does not go away.

I field these "weight gain, belly fat" calls on a daily basis. Women who call me are complaining about 2 things"

1) A weight gain of between 10-40 pounds. Yes, I am not joking, and I am sure many of you are sadly nodding in agreement.
2) The change in the shape of their bodies. You ask, "What is going on?" You have new fat accumulated around your stomach area. Somehow, this might be easier to take if it was evenly distributed over your entire body. Instead, you have pants that don't fit, zippers left undone and you are investing in tunic tops. SPANX is the new Wall Street darling because we are all struggling.

Well, I've got great news for you. There is a solution. It is NOT about your willpower. It is NOT about fasting and starving. It is NOT about exercising. NO....it is about your HORMONES. Accumulation of belly fat is a tell-tale signal of hormone imbalance.

Hormones control weight gain, weight distribution, where you store your fat, and also your metabolism. Hormones even control your appetite and cravings. If you are unbalanced in any way, your efforts will be sabotaged, and you will fail…no matter how hard you diet and how much you exercise.

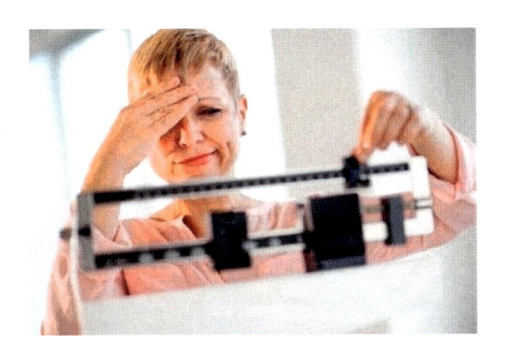

FACT: As we age, hormones steadily decline in both women AND men and easily become imbalanced. You can quickly find excess weight accumulating in your abdomen.

Your abdomen may become so distended that you appear pregnant.

This type of fat accumulation can begin very early. I have seen teens with this body distortion.

And then we become miserable, worried, and even depressed. What happened to our body?

Friends, we are out of balance! Hormone balance.

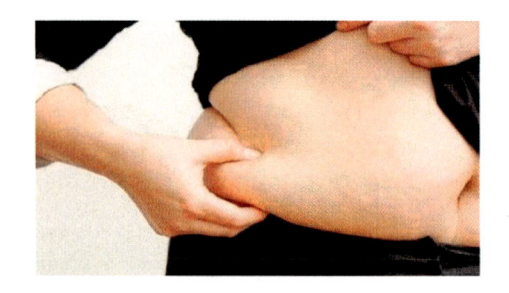

Hormone imbalance between estrogen, progesterone, cortisol, insulin, DHEA, melatonin, and testosterone will cause that belly fat to settle in, become almost "nuclear" and be nearly impossible to lose despite your best efforts.

Besides being annoying to you from an appearance standpoint, belly and abdominal fat increase your risk of obesity, diabetes and heart disease. Abdominal fat needs to GO!

The Solution: You can restore your hormone balance and eliminate those pounds that are sitting right there in your middle.

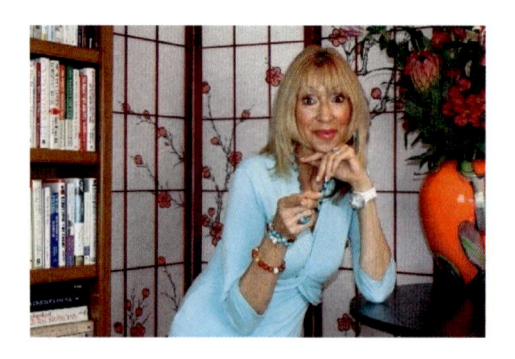

"Balance Your Hormones, Balance Your Life!"

THE GOOD NEWS:

I can help you restore your HORMONE BALANCE! I also have some great suggestions for supplements that will help you in your quest which we will discuss in a bit. Success can start within a week or so. Now I want you to give it time but you can lose 1 to 2 inches off your waist line in the first few weeks. By the second month you'll notice even better results as your metabolism picks up and burns that stubborn belly fat You can change the way you look AND shock your scale!

With Hormone Balance: Your FAT STORAGE ZONE becomes your FAT BURNING ZONE

The Genesis:

Why did that belly fat appear in the first place? Generally, in women it is due to the current "estrogen dominance" epidemic. There are so many environmental estrogens that are attacking you daily and your body can quickly become overwhelmed. I have seen women begin to pack on the pounds in their early to mid 30's and by age 50 they have gained 10-40 unwanted pounds.

This weight goes right around the middle and can be almost impossible to lose <u>UNTIL HORMONES ARE BALANCED.</u>

Restricting calories will not work. Our metabolism slows as we approach menopause. Calorie restriction lowers metabolism even more. So it is very difficult to lose those extra pounds simply by restricting calories. Dieting can be a losing battle and very frustrating. Many of you call me in tears.

Natural hormones are key. We need to decrease estrogen dominance, increase progesterone, regulate cortisol, keep DHEA levels healthy, increase melatonin, and keep thyroid normal. This can all be done naturally.

WHY NATURAL HORMONES?

Many physicians ignore natural hormones. In medical school most doctors are not educated about the benefits. They receive most of their information from studies funded by the pharmaceutic companies. Natural hormones are not patentable because they are not altered chemically and do not produce any profits for the drug companies. Pharmaceutical companies do not tell you about studies that compare synthetic hormones vs natural hormones because those studies would not be favorable.

Natural hormones work to restore hormone balance, and they are safer and more effective than drug alternatives. Can man create a better hormone than one derived from nature? No. In fact, many medical schools are now incorporating the study of natural hormones in their curriculums. The wheels are turning! Natural hormones can reverse your Belly Fat. Synthetics can contribute to your Belly Fat.

Another note: You will undoubtedly encounter a "Saboteur" as you go along with the Belly Flat program. They will tell you that you will not succeed. Seriously, be prepared. I have seen it over and over, even among my closest friends.

"Misery loves company", as my mother would say. They don't want to do the work and they don't want you to do it either.

Please don't let a saboteur stop you. You can do it!

Now, we are going to get technical as we go along: I encourage you to highlight the passages that relate to you as you go through the book. And remember, you can always email me. I promise to answer! barbara@askbarbarahoffman.com

WATCH OUT FOR ESTROGEN: Countless women are put on estrogen by their doctors even when it is not estrogen, but progesterone that they need. And estrogen is the fat STORAGE hormone. Did you know you make estrogen in your fat cells? That means you're making it all of your life.

The "Catch 22" is that the more estrogen you have, the more fat you store and the more fat cells you make. So now you have more fat cells that want to produce and store more estrogen. Your body has now become a fat magnet! It's the proverbial vicious cycle. So, obviously, estrogen is not the answer.

Progesterone balances estrogen. Progesterone is the hormone that you essentially stop making once you stop ovulating, so in perimenopause and menopause most women are progesterone DEFICIENT. Even if you are still menstruating, if you are not ovulating, you are not making progesterone.

HERE IS WHAT WOMEN ARE SAYING

"I am 51 years old and have had no waist line for quite some time! I always felt bloated and sluggish. I discovered that I was low in progesterone. I have used progesterone crème for 6 months now and my waist line is back. I can feel my body going down every day. Also, my energy is rising! I have lost 12 pounds in the last 6 months and I have not changed my eating habits. I know it is the progesterone. I am not feeling so bloated and swollen and the muffin top is gone! My clothes look good on me again"
- Melinda B.

"I have lost 14 pounds in the past 6 months and I have not changed my eating habits. I know it is the progesterone. I'm not feeling bloated and swollen and my clothes look so good on me." – Victoria S.

THIS CAN BE YOU

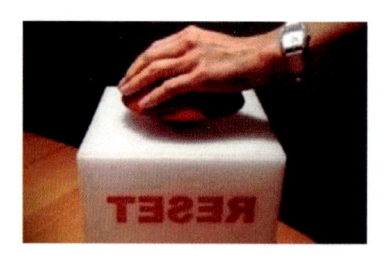

HORMONE RESET

With Belly Fat you need to figure out exactly where your imbalance originates.
There are 7 culprits to watch for.
Here is an overview. We will address each one of these individually.

- **High Estrogen**
- **High Insulin**
- **High Cortisol**
- **Low Progesterone**
- **Low DHEA**
- **Low Melatonin**
- **Low Thyroid**
- **Low Testosterone**

Onward we go…. towards hormone balance and no more Belly Fat!

Chapter 2
Estrogen Dominance

KEY POINT: When the ratio of estrogen to progesterone is out of balance, your entire body can become a "fat magnet!"

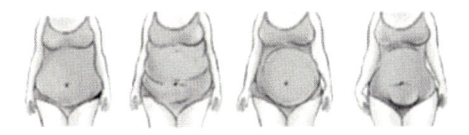

Women: High Estrogen = Belly Fat. Estrogen dominance controls your body's fat distribution. Instead of the body storing any extra calories evenly over legs, arms, neck, face, estrogen tells the body to store the fat right around the abdomen or midsection. That is why we women end up with the "pooch" (and the men end up with the "spare tire").

Men: are you lethargic, getting increased breast tissue? Do you have a belly that looks like a "beer belly?" Abdominal fat in men increases the conversion of testosterone into estrogen. As estrogen levels rise, so does the tendency to accumulate more abdominal fat, fueling the situation. The risk of prostate cancer also increases with higher estrogen levels. So men would be wise to oppose excess estrogens with progesterone.

IMPORTANT: when you are estrogen dominant your body will stubbornly REFUSE to use stored fat for energy. Instead of burning the fat, your body says "store, store, store…We might need this fat later." Estrogen becomes a bully. No matter how much you exercise or how much you diet, that estrogen will not let you burn the fat that has now been stored around your middle.

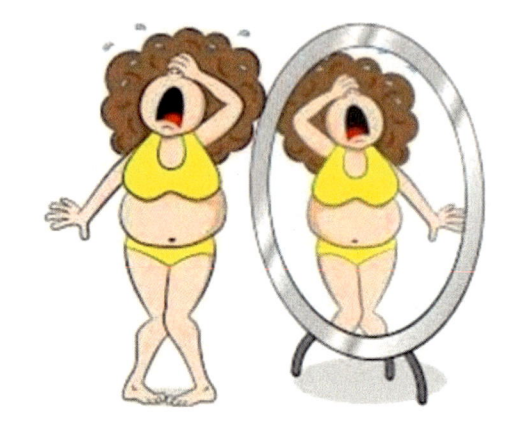

"Help me!"

You ask, "How do I become estrogen dominant? I thought my estrogen levels were dropping as I got older?" Yes, they do drop. But all hormones drop with age. What you want to look at is the RATIO between estrogen and progesterone. Simply said, if your estrogen is too high in relationship to your progesterone, you are estrogen dominant, no matter how low your estrogen is.

DOES DIETING WORK?

Let's talk diet...Are you eating the same foods but now you pooch up? So now you're dieting, eating celery & carrots and fasting and the pooch is still there? Well, that is the infamous "estrogen dominance belly fat." Unfortunately, dieting won't solve the issue.

Key Symptoms of Estrogen Dominance:

- Weight Gain around the mid-section
- Overall weight gain
- Bloating / fluid retention
- Insomnia, restless sleep
- Fatigue
- Memory loss / Inability to concentrate
- Menstrual cramps
- Irregular menstrual flow
- Depression
- Thyroid imbalance/hypothyroid
- Anxiety / Panic attacks
- Inability to concentrate
- Osteoporosis, osteopenia
- Cold hands and feet
- Breast tenderness
- Decreased mental sharpness
- Mood swings / Irritability
- Heavy periods
- Hair Loss
- Fibrocystic breast disease
- Uterine fibroids
- Loss of sexual desire
- Acne
- Dry Eyes
- Clotting
- Urinary frequency

SUPPLEMENTS:

DIM (Diindolylmethane) –
 detoxes excess estrogen
Vitex – promotes estrogen / progesterone
 balance
Progesterone – opposes excess estrogen.
 The "Balancing Hormone"

You may need an estrogen detox.
See chapter 10

Chapter 3
Insulin Resistance

KEY POINT: For a Flat Belly, it is vital to keep your insulin LOW

Insulin is an important hormone which is essential to process all sugar that enters our body. Insulin aids the bloodstream to carry glucose into our cells...There it is either used as fuel (as gasoline in a car) OR stored as fat. Insulin can become a "Bully" if you consume too much sugar. The higher your blood glucose after consumption of food, the greater your insulin level and the MORE FAT IS DEPOSITED! This fat deposition is especially visible in the abdomen. Then, the bigger your belly, the poorer your response to insulin since the deep visceral fat of the belly is associated with resistance to insulin which I show in the graphic below.

HOW DOES INSULIN WORK?

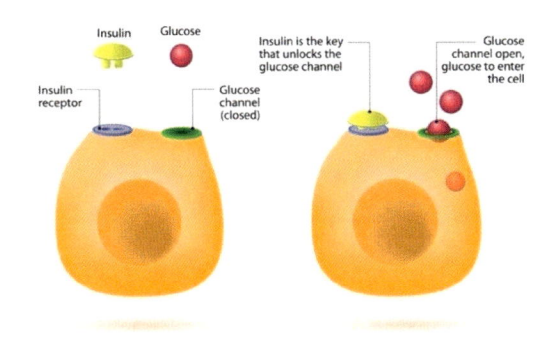

When your insulin levels are consistently high, you will develop a condition called Insulin Resistance. This is also known as "metabolic syndrome" A shocking fact: 1 of every 4 Americans has insulin resistance. That is why we see so much belly fat!!

IR IN A NUTSHELL:

You Eat

⬇

Glucose Goes To The Cells for Storage

⬇

Insulin Opens Cell Doors

⬇

High Insulin (too many carbs) – Cell doors close to the glucose

⬇

Glucose ends up being stored in the wrong areas

⬇

The Result: STORED FAT!

What to do: Restrict SUGAR and CARBS. This is the best thing you can do for yourself. First, sugar is not your friend as far as insulin is concerned. I think we all know that, but sugar is so tempting. Do not succumb if you want to lose the Belly Fat.

CARBS: Carbs activate insulin because so many carbs convert to sugar and tell your body to <u>hang on to existing fat and to even store more fat.</u> "Oh no," you say. "I love my potatoes, pasta, bread" These are all carbs and carbs can be "bullies", just like estrogen and insulin.

If you truly want to lose the Belly Fat, you are going to take a Carb Break until you get the flat belly back again.

You can still eat! I am not a diet fan…I like to see you eat. Did you know? Proteins and fats need to be broken down before being turned into glucose and this takes time.

Your body has to work harder to digest them. So protein and fat do NOT give you an insulin spike. Go ahead and have that meatball, that avocado, those nuts and even that cheese if you like cheese. You will not be raising your insulin level.

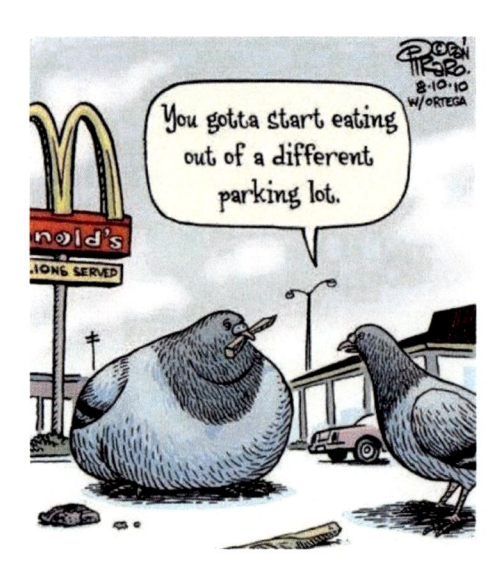

Do not skip meals! Skipping meals makes your liver less sensitive to insulin and will prompt your body to store calories as fat instead of burning them. So eat 3 meals per day and include snacks (healthy, of course!)

Protein stimulates the hormones that control appetite. It ALSO helps your body burn fat. A study published in *Diabetes Care* compared a high-protein diet with a low-protein diet in men and women with type 2 diabetes. Those on the high-protein diet had significantly greater reductions in abdominal fat. Also, a greater reduction in LDL ("bad") cholesterol.

Important: Bump up your protein, including in snacks. Higher protein keeps your blood sugar in balance and insulin levels low. It will also help with appetite control and fat burning.

Need some help with choosing great proteins?
Best suggestions are: chicken, turkey, low fat cheese and hard-boiled eggs. If you like fish, that's even better.

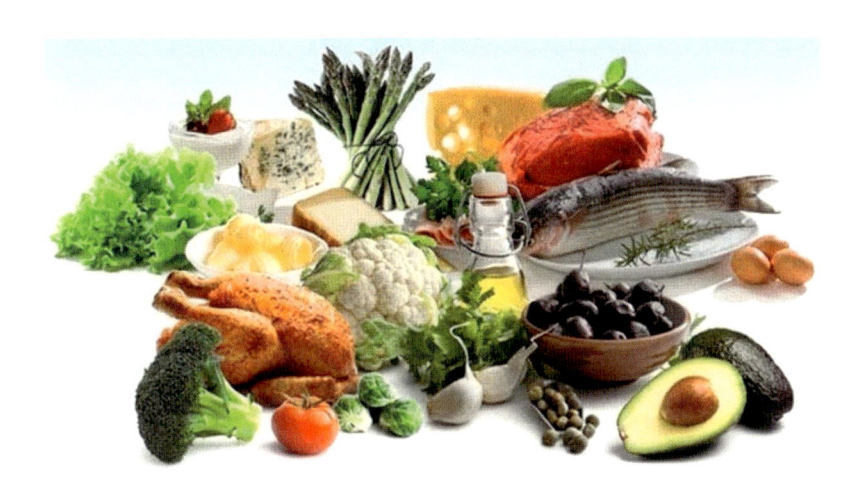

Need more help?
I invite you to visit my Eat Your Self Slender page for snack and meal suggestions.

http://www.bhnformulas.com/eyss-home-page.html

SUGAR:

Sugar has GOT to go! Sugar is notorious for raising insulin and blocking fat metabolism. It can also block thyroid function.

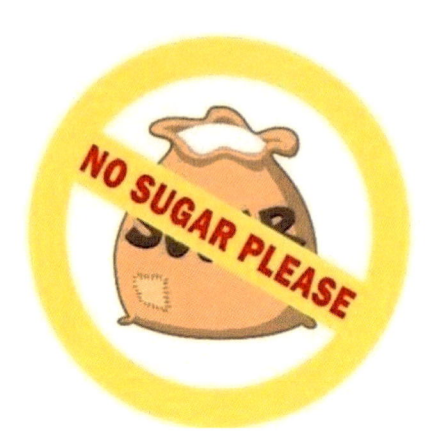

Stick to 20 grams of sugar per meal and 15 - 20 grams per snack. Read the labels. I've been doing this for years and sometimes I am SHOCKED at how many sugar grams are in something that looks "healthy" ...like a protein bar for instance. Be vigilant.

Having a hard time thinking of giving up sugar?

At the end of this book, I have my 6-part get off sugar program. I will EASE you thru it!

Chapter 4
High Insulin Recap

KEY POINT: High insulin is your Belly Flat enemy. It can be a "silent saboteur"

Key Symptoms of High Insulin

Weight Gain in the hips / thigh area

Hair loss

Anxiety

Difficulty concentrating

PCOS – Polycystic Ovarian Syndrome

Acne

Cravings for sugary and high-carb foods

Intense/Frequent Hunger

SUPPLEMENTS:

ChromeMate – helps keep blood sugar normal

PGX – helps keep blood sugar normal

Magnesium – can lower fasting blood sugar levels

Chromium – combats high insulin

Chapter 5
High Cortisol

High Cortisol: ("The Stress Hormone") Makes you feel hungry all the time!

KEY POINT: Your body is not able to deal with consistently high levels of cortisol. High cortisol increases appetite and cravings. You will be hungrier, feel more cravings and struggle with bingeing. You will always reach for the chips, not the carrots!

High Cortisol promotes High Insulin which translates to Belly Fat.

Elevated cortisol causes abdominal fat. High cortisol ALSO increases appetite and cravings. You brain gets the "eat-store" signal, just as with high estrogen. Also, high cortisol leads to lower testosterone because when you are stressed, your body will make cortisol instead of testosterone.

So we become untoned, soft and flabby. Even if you are thin, like me, you can get belly fat if you have high cortisol because you are *storing, storing, storing* fat. Another sign of high cortisol is "Back Fat"

Yes, cortisol is essential to us because it helps the body use sugar (glucose) and fat for energy (metabolism), and it helps the body manage stress.

BUT elevated levels are deadly to our health AND to our body shape. Cortisol is known as the "Stress Hormone" and it serves a useful purpose to get us through times of need. But if you have more stress than normal, feel exhausted all the time, or have anxiety, you may very likely have high cortisol.

The cortisol mechanism: Normal cortisol should follow a specific biorhythm during the day. If at any time during the day you have an excess release of cortisol it will affect both your **blood sugar and your insulin secretion**.

Circadian rhythm and your cortisol cycle

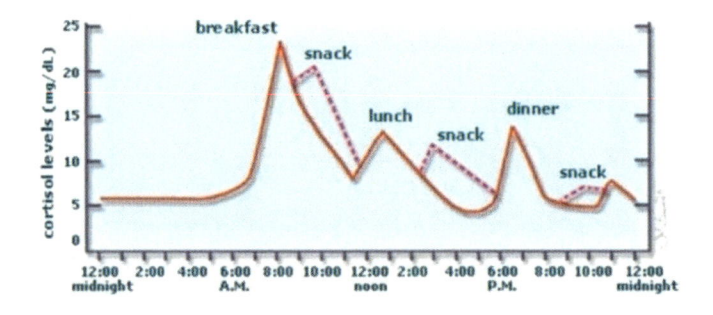

The cortisol rhythm is tied to our sleep / wake pattern. Levels should be highest when we first wake up in the morning. Light hits our eyes and a signal is sent out that the day has begun. Adrenalin begins to pump and the cortisol helps us wake up from our slumber.

Normally, cortisol levels begin to drop later in the morning, but as morning turns to afternoon they begin to rise again. The highest point is right around the middle of the day. When cortisol is high, metabolism increases and we receive a signal that it is time to eat.

So you can see, if cortisol levels are <u>always</u> high, you are <u>always</u> hungry.

As we head into evening, cortisol should decrease and your body prepare for rest. Melatonin begins to secrete and you get the "time to end the day and rest" signal.

This cycle is very important! You do not want a disrupted cortisol rhythm!

"Why would my cortisol be elevated?"

Here is a check list: Family or relationship stress, family illness, the death of a loved one, divorce, loss of a job, financial obligations, moving, chronic illness, anger, guilt, depression, anxiety, taking care of an elderly or sick family member, a traumatic event, too much caffeine (which I consider to be over 4 cups of coffee per day…I love coffee! But no more than 4 cups per day), insufficient sleep and overstimulation with computer screens or TV.

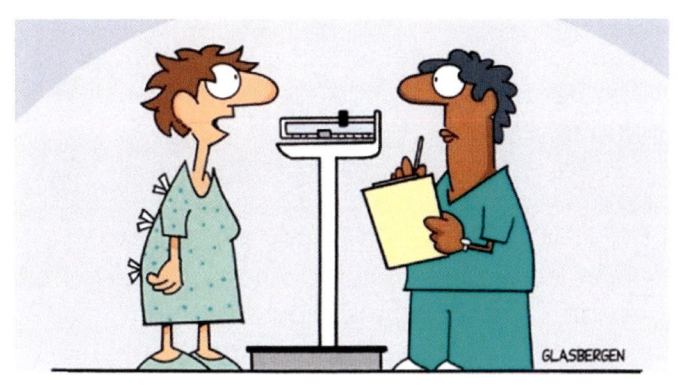

"I'm a wife, a mother, a daughter, an executive, a cook, a housekeeper, a teacher, a chauffeur, and a soccer coach. That's only 19 pounds per woman!"

The Good News: Lowering cortisol can help you:

Eliminate the "Muffin Top"
Reduce nighttime hunger
Reduce sugar cravings
Improve Sleep quality

Cortisol Balancing Tips:

Sleep 7-9 hours per night to reduce stress.
Eat a high protein breakfast within 1 hour of getting out of bed.
Do not go longer than 3 hours between snacks and meals.

SUPPLEMENTS:

Phosphatidylserine: 100 mg per day. PS will detoxify and break down excess cortisol to get you back to normal. Cortisol receptors get damaged by high cortisol levels. PS helps repair the feedback control apparatus and can correct high cortisol levels. I love it and take it daily.

Rhodiola Rosea: 500 mg per day. Rhodiola also helps restore cortisol balance. It is an adaptogen that helps the adrenal glands produce cortisol in NORMAL patterns. There is also a wonderful extract that I love if you don't like taking pills. I will list it at the back in the supplements section. You can take it whenever you are feeling immediately stressed.

Wondering about your cortisol levels? Remember, they should be high in the morning and low at night. A simple saliva test can determine your cortisol biorhythm for the day. A good home test can be found at [www.zrtlabs.com.](www.zrtlabs.com) They will mail the test kit directly to you, you collect the saliva specimen and mail it back to them. Within 7-10 days you will have your test results.

Chapter 6

Low Progesterone

KEY POINT: Progesterone is the "master balancer" of all the hormones

Estrogen dominance is opposed
Insulin release is regulated
It enhances the production of thyroid hormone
It enhances the production of thyroid hormone
It acts as a natural diuretic, reducing bloating
Can support melatonin levels for good sleep
Helps keep serotonin at normal levels to control appetite, cravings & binge eating.

Progesterone is your "Flat Belly" best friend hormone. I would start here. I can't be more emphatic.

Progesterone OPPOSES the estrogen dominance that will cause you to store fat in the midsection. Progesterone causes the food you eat to be BURNED for energy instead of being stored as FAT! This is known as thermogenesis.

It is a truly remarkable hormone. Progesterone will kickstart your weight loss at the cellular level AND it helps your thyroid stay healthy. <u>Bonus: when progesterone and estrogen are balanced, blood sugar levels are encouraged to remain normal and you will not have obsessive cravings.</u>

Symptoms of Low Progesterone:

- Insomnia
- Water Retention
- Irritability / Mood Swings
- Depression
- Irregular Menstrual Cycle
- Uterine Fibroids
- Breast Tenderness
- Anxiety
- Low libido
- Fatigue
- Weight gain / sugar cravings
- Hair Loss
- Muscle Pains
- PCOS
- Endometriosis
- Slow metabolism
- Acne
- Vaginal Dryness
- Infertility
- Ovarian Cysts

These symptoms may sound common to some of you, **but they are not normal.** If you have any of these symptoms, it is essential to get your hormones back in balance as soon as you can. The symptoms usually will get worse as time goes on, especially the weight gain.

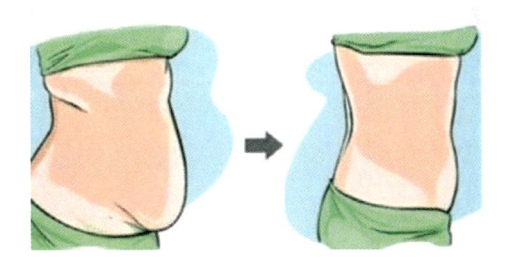

Victory with progesterone!

Crème or Pill?
The best, most efficient way, to use progesterone is a transdermal crème. You get the full dose that you actually use because liver metabolism is not involved. The progesterone proceeds directly to the receptor sites. With the crème version, your body actually thinks it made the progesterone in your ovaries and the response is immediate. With oral progesterone (pills) you involve the liver and ultimately only get 10-20% of the dose. So…doctors prescribe 200 mg to give you 20 mg. Oral progesterone side effects include drowsiness, constipation, and BLOATING…is exactly what we are trying to avoid.

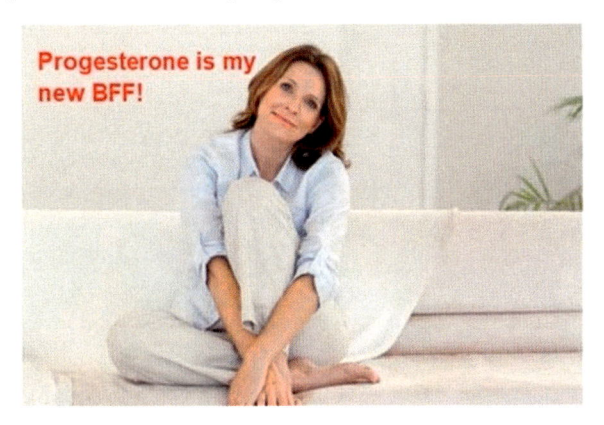

Note: Even low estrogen levels can result in estrogen dominance if your body is not producing progesterone every month. You can see, then, during peri-menopause and menopause even when your estrogen levels drop, estrogen dominance can still be a big problem. You are making no progesterone, but you still make enough estrogen, in your fat cells. Estrogen levels never decline to zero, but progesterone can. So...progesterone to the rescue!

You do not need a prescription for transdermal progesterone. Look for one that contains 1000 mg of micronized progesterone per 2 ounce jar. Also, look for one that does not contain parabens or too many extracurricular ingredients. The purer, the better.

Warning: Do not use synthetic progestins, as found in birth control pills. They can <u>cause</u> Belly Fat. They are "no-no's in the most serious sense. They do not sit properly on our hormone receptor sites, so the body gets confused and sends them to other areas of the body to try and fit in. So they wreak hormone havoc. Also, synthetic doses are much higher that the percentage our body usually makes. No wonder they pack on the pounds!

- ❖ Think you have excess estrogen? We will discuss estrogen detox in a bit. You will prevail!

Chapter 7
Low DHEA

Key point: DHEA declines rapidly after the age of 40. It is considered by experts to be a potent weapon in the "Battle of the Bulge"

Symptoms of low DHEA

- Belly Fat, weight gain, obesity,
- Extreme fatigue even if you have slept 8 hours
- Moodiness
- Decrease in muscle mass
- Depression
- Aching joints
- Low libido
- Lack of vaginal lubrication/dryness
- Hypothyroidism
- Loss in bone mineral density

DHEA is a bio-identical hormone that is produced in your adrenal glands. You may have heard it called the "Fountain of Youth" because of its anti-aging effects. DHEA levels peak at age 20 and then decline as we age. So, if you are over the age of 45 you are most probably low in DHEA.

DHEA LOWERS AS WE AGE

How does DHEA help with Belly Fat?

DHEA enhances the thermogenic process of food, meaning food is transferred into energy <u>instead of fat.</u> People taking DHEA experienced significant losses in visceral and subcutaneous fat. Women lost an average of 10.2% of their belly fat and men lost an average of 7.4%. DHEA also helps you regain muscle mass which increases fat burning.

I find that DHEA helps me feel youthful, energetic and motivated to face my day. It can also boost libido, if that is of interest to you.

DHEA Supplements

I like a dose of 10-20 mg for a woman and 25-50 mg for a man. Do not go overboard and take excess. Stick with the normal physiologic dose. Remember, our goal is to stay <u>in balance</u>.

Chapter 8
Low Melatonin

Key point: This is our "Sleep Hormone". When you go into deep sleep, hormones are reset, released and re-balanced. Melatonin lowers cortisol.

Symptoms of Low Melatonin
- Difficulty falling asleep at night
- Awakening during the night and having difficulty getting back to sleep
- Waking very early in the morning without being able to get back to sleep.
- Restless sleep
- Feeling unrefreshed in the morning
- Lack of dreams
- Fatigue. Confusion or forgetfulness
- Depressed mood

My friends, sleep is extremely important to our Flat Belly Plan. We need a good solid 7-9 hours per night. Why? Poor sleep causes us to wake up too high in cortisol, which we have discussed is the stress hormone. Overly high cortisol in the morning fuels appetite and cravings ALL DAY LONG!
So, we start out disadvantaged before we even put our foot on the floor. AND, worst of all, we will crave sugar and carbs. Good sleep keeps our belly FLAT because the sleep hormone melatonin helps control our appetite and also increases metabolism.

Good sleep promotes appetite control. It boosts leptin. Leptin is the hormone that tells us to "put down the fork" after we have eaten enough. If you are getting only 5 hours of sleep per night, you will get belly fat in spite of diet and exercise. So... you need your "shut eye". Did you ever wonder why God designed us to sleep for 8 hours per night when He could have let us go active 24-7? Because we need to restore ourselves during sleep! So, let's get sleeping.

You need 5 cycles of sleep each night. Each cycle takes 90 minutes. 5 x 90 minutes = 7 ½ hours. To determine your bedtime, take the time you need or want to be up in the morning and count back 7 ½ hours. Then go to sleep at that hour.

If you are having problems, melatonin is for you.

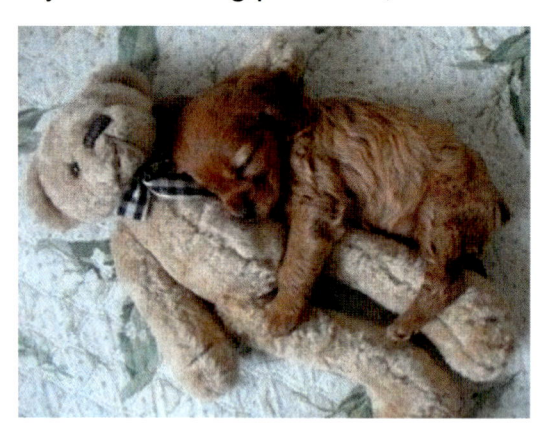

How does it work?
Melatonin is not a sleeping pill. It is a hormone. It will reset your circadian rhythm back to normal. It can take from 1 - 6 weeks to accomplish this.

A sleeping pill, like Ambien or Lunesta, will NOT restore normal sleep cycles, when you discontinue sleeping pills, insomnia returns.

Take Melatonin about 45 Minutes to 1 hour before you plan to sleep. Begin with a dose of 1 milligram. I personally take 5 mg per night, but I started with 1 mg. You can take additional melatonin if you repeatedly wake up during the night, using the supplement to create a deeper sleep, but give it a try for a week or so before moving to a higher dose.

- *Watch for any side effects the next day. If you feel groggy, you can take the melatonin earlier in the evening.*
- *Expect some vivid dreams for the first week. This is a good thing—a sign you are in deep sleep.*

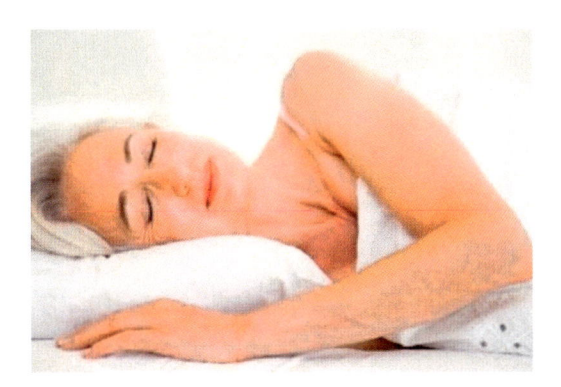

Chapter 9
Low Thyroid

KEY POINT

Hormone imbalance, especially estrogen dominance, negatively affects your thyroid. The thyroid has a metabolic function that helps our bodies maintain a normal weight. With estrogen dominance, the estrogen becomes a bully to the thyroid and will actually "beat up" the thyroid gland so thyroid function and metabolism slow down. So…the bane of our existence…More Fat Storage!
Sugar can also inflame and damage thyroid function! See my 6 part Get Off Sugar series on page 90

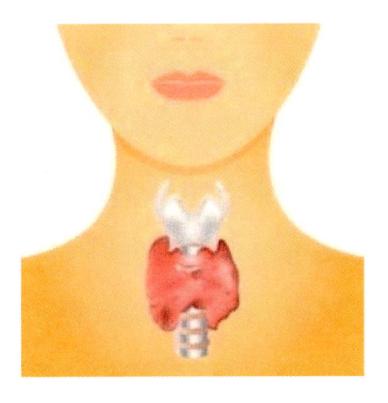

If your body were a bus, your thyroid would be the gas pedal.

SYMPTOMS OF LOW THYROID:

Extreme fatigue
Hair loss
Outer 1/3 of your eyebrows is missing
Cold hands, feet
Dry brittle hair
Dry skin
Dry, gritty eyes
Poor Immune System

Eating more of the following foods that are rich in iodine may help you boost your thyroid function:
- Low-fat cheese
- Eggs
- Yogurt
- Saltwater fish
- Seaweed (including kelp, dulce, nori)
- Shellfish

Important: SOY INHIBITS THYROID
Be careful with soy products. In recent years soy has become enormously popular, due to the reports that Asian women have less reported breast cancer than Western women.

However, processed soy is not the answer! Processed soy products have been shown to reduce the conversion of the thyroid hormone T4 to T3. In a recent study, daily soy consumption resulted in symptoms of hypothyroidism in 50% of human subjects tested.

Note: Fermented soy products (miso, tempeh, tofu) did not have the negative effect. THESE are the products consumed by Asian women, not the processed soy products such as soy nuts and soy nutrition bars.

SUPPLEMENTS:

Natural progesterone: remember Progesterone is "best friends" with your thyroid.
L-Tyrosine: A lack of tyrosine in the diet may lead to an underactive thyroid
Iodine
Selenium: helps convert T4 to T3
DHEA: A good overall over-all thyroid supplement

Are you sensing how all the hormones work together? Let's keep going! No Belly Fat for us!

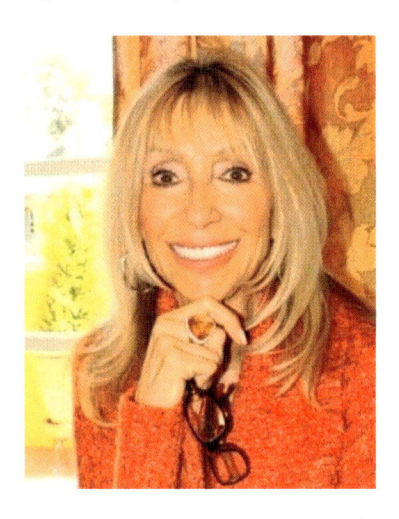

Chapter 10

Low Testosterone

Key Point: If you have low testosterone, you are more likely to develop a "pot belly" and other body fat.

Symptoms of low Testosterone in Women
- Fatigue & Exhaustion
- Weight gain & difficulty losing weight
- Decreased interest in sex
- Depressed mood.
- Lethargy.
- Muscle weakness.

Symptoms of low Testosterone in Men
- Low sex drive
- Feeling numb in the genital area
- Fatigue / Decreased Energy
- Feeling blue; no optimism
- Muscle weakness.
- Decreased interest in sex

How does Testosterone help reduce Belly Fat?

People with low testosterone are more likely to develop a "pot belly" and other body fat. Also, your muscle mass decreases which leads to even more flab.

SUPPLEMENTS:

DHEA increases testosterone levels. So, if you cannot get a prescription for testosterone, this is a great supplement for you.

Tribulus terrestris can raise testosterone by reducing the binding of testosterone to the sex hormone binding globulin (SHBG). So your testosterone remains "free" to be utilized by your body.

Chapter 11
Estrogen Detox

ESTROGEN DETOX WILL HELP REDUCE/ELIMINATE BELLY FAT

70% of women 50 years of age and older report that they are trying unsuccessfully to lose weight. "Estrogen weight" can be almost nuclear! An estrogen detox is key. You want to OPTIMIZE estrogen metabolism and DETOX excess estrogen.

You ask...WHAT DO I DO? I think I need the Estrogen Detox. Yes, a detox can work wonders. There is a remarkable supplement that can do the trick for you in just 3 months!
But first, a quick lesson: There are 2 estrogen "pathways" thru which estrogen is metabolized.

The 2-hydroxy pathway results in beneficial, or "good," estrogen metabolites.
The "bad" estrogen metabolism pathway is the 16-hydroxy pathway. Estrogen broken down in this pathway results in metabolites responsible for many of estrogen's undesirable actions, including weight gain.

What is the detox supplement?

DIM (diindolylmethane, pronounced: dye-indollmethane).
DIM shifts estrogen metabolism to the 2-hydroxy pathway, resulting in healthier estrogen metabolites and restored hormonal balance. DIM acts like a "traffic cop," guiding used estrogen down the 2-hydroxy pathway and promoting healthy estrogen metabolism in men and women. DIM increases the body's natural ability to burn fat!

DIM is a phytochemical naturally found in small amounts in cruciferous vegetables such as cabbage, cauliflower, and broccoli, but you'd have to eat a couple of heads of broccoli to get the same dose as an easy-to-swallow nutritional supplement.

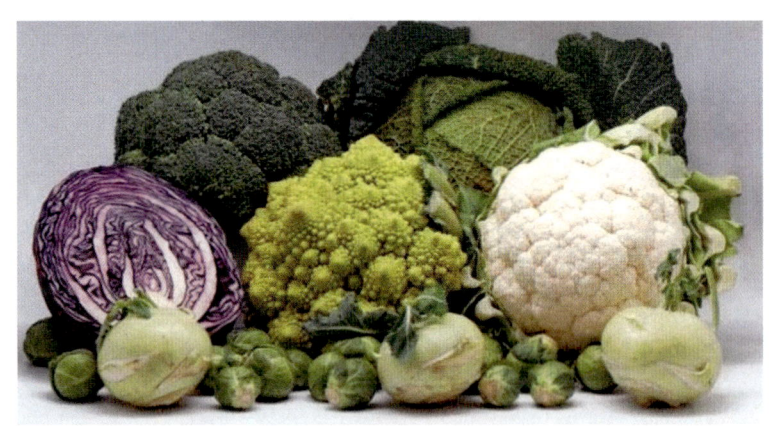

Can't eat all this? DIM to the rescue!

How does it work? When you turn your estrogen onto the "good" pathway, your body will release stored fat. No more "Estrogen Belly"

When you take DIM, the excess estrogen passes thru the stool and out of the body. Gone!

Another thing I love about DIM…It acts to stimulate serotonin production which contributes to our emotional well-being, enhances mood and suppresses appetite by stimulating serotonin production.

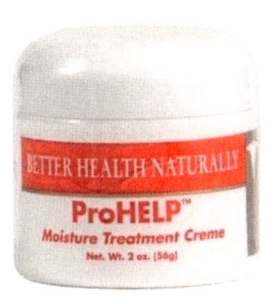

Also, you know by now, if you are one of my followers, that Progesterone pushes Estrogen to a good mode of storage, not allowing the bad metabolites. So don't forget your progesterone crème!

I personally take DIM for 3 months, STOP for 2 months and then repeat the cycle.

Foods to Avoid to keep Estrogen balanced

Top 5 Estrogenic Foods You Must Avoid

Soy

Soy mimics estrogen and so has the same effect as estrogen on the body. Eating soy daily can push you into estrogen dominance. Fermented products are fine. These are Miso, Tempeh, & Tofu. These are your soy "friends".

Sugar

This should not be a Surprise! Simple carbohydrates raise estrogen. Stay away from white rice, white-bread, and pasta. Fat cells LOVE carbs and sugar. Think of it this way, you are FEEDING your fat cells.

Meat

The high levels of estrogen in certain red meat is actually causing girls to enter puberty at younger ages, around 10-12 instead of 13-17. That's how powerful the effect of hormone-laden meat is. If you eat meat or serve meat to your family, choose beef that has not been fed hormones!

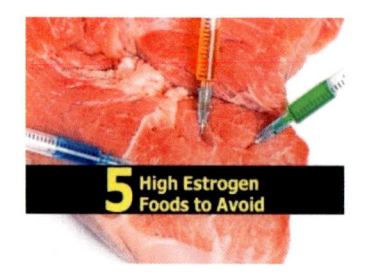

Dairy

Cow dairy contains 20 different chemicals that affect hormone levels in the body. Choose goat milk products instead. OR choose Almond Milk or Cashew Milk.

BPA

Plastic bottles containing BPA should never be left in the sun or heated. Teflon pans are another culprit of high estrogen—when heated, they emit 400x more PFOAs.

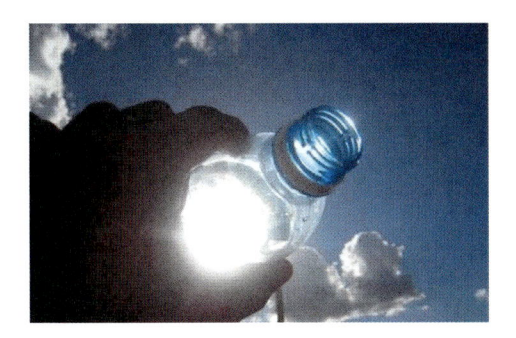

Foods that Actually Detox Estrogen

These foods are your Belly Flat BFF's!

1.) Indole-3 Carbinole (found in cruciferous vegetables) If you cut any of these vegetables, you will see a sign of the cross…hence, cruciferous, meaning "cross". Eat them in abundance.

- Broccoli
- Cauliflower
- Celery
- Cabbage
- Kale
- Brussels sprouts
- Bok Choy

The cruciferous vegetables provide powerful estrogen-protecting compounds, known as glucoraphanin and di-indoly methane (DIM) that promote excess estrogen elimination via the C-2 pathway.

2.) Sesame and flax: These unique seeds provide a special type of fiber called lignans, which can bind to estrogen in the digestive tract so that it will be readily excreted from the body. These seeds also increase levels of SHGB (sex hormone binding globulin), which protects the body from estrogen, while simultaneously improving balance of all hormones.

3.) Salmon & Oily Fish. The omega-3 fats, EPA and DHA, which are found in fish, help the body eliminate estrogen safely down a pathway that doesn't damage DNA or cause cancer. Additionally, fish oil has an inflammation-fighting effect, while also improving insulin signaling for a healthier metabolism.

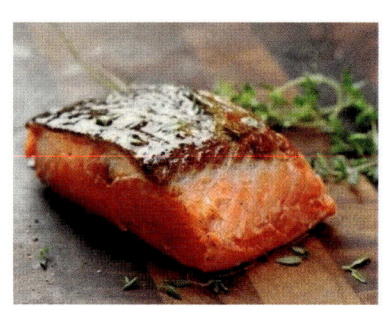

4.) Lemon & Citrus Fruits. Lemons and the other citrus fruits provide antioxidants (vitamin, hesperidin, and quercetin) that protect against damage from estrogen. They are also rich in fiber which promotes good elimination. Best of all, citrus are packed with the compound D-limonene, which modulates liver enzymes so that the body is better able to metabolize and remove estrogen.

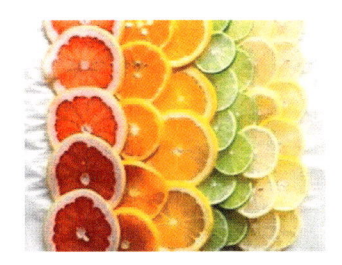

5.) Yogurt & Other Fermented Foods. Foods that contain healthy probiotic bacteria can help reduce body fat so you get less estrogen secretion from your fat cells. They are also helpful for excess estrogen elimination. Examples of good probiotic foods are Greek yogurt, sauerkraut, pickled ginger, kimchi, and miso.

6.) Green Tea. Since green tea can boost the metabolic rate, it can help you lose weight. Studies show that green tea leads to decreases in body fat, body weight, waist circumference and abdominal fat (the "Belly Fat") Women who drink more green tea have lower breast cancer rates due to the powerful anti-aromatase action in tea. Thus, less estrogen is synthesized from testosterone. Excess estrogen is NOT desirable as we have discussed.

7.) High-Protein Foods. Protein is necessary for the activity of cytochrome P450, which are enzymes that allow the body to metabolize excess hormones from the body. High protein foods such as fish, meat, beans, and eggs also provide the amino acids lysine and theonine that support liver function, which is the organ that is ultimately responsible for safely eliminating estrogen from the body.

Chapter 12
Boost Your Fat Burners For Lasting Success

1) Increase Metabolism

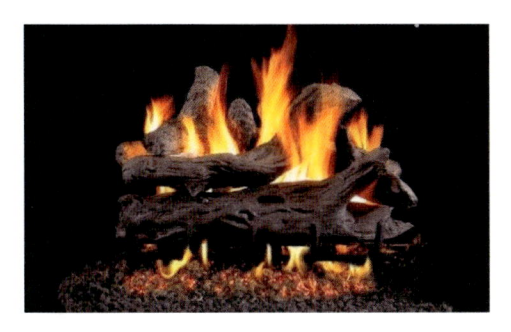

Your metabolism is like a fire – you want flames, not just glowing embers that don't increase metabolism.

1. **ALWAYS REV UP IN THE MORNING**:
   Eating breakfast jump-starts metabolism and keeps energy high all day. Women who skip breakfast are 4 1/2 times as likely to be obese. If nothing else, grab a yogurt. I personally like ½ of a chicken breast in the morning, a couple of slices of deli honey-roast turkey, or 2 hard-boiled eggs with a little mayo.
   I have some good high protein breakfast ideas in my book, *Eat Yourself Slender*, if you would like more help.

2. EAT ENOUGH:
Cutting calories to a too-low level delivers a double whammy to your metabolism. You eat less and your body shuts down to preserve fat for energy. It also begins to break down precious, calorie-burning muscle tissue for energy You have just "put the brakes" on your metabolism. This is NOT the way to go. Make sure to have your snacks midmorning and midafternoon between meals to keep your metabolism humming along.

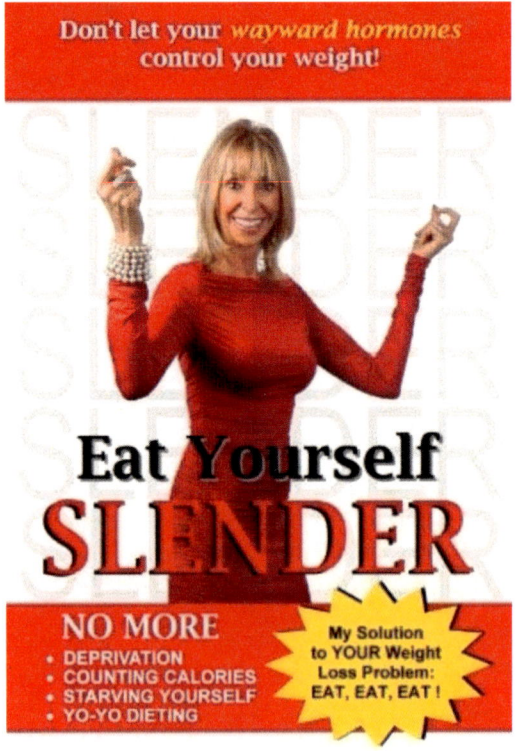

Don't let your *wayward hormones* control your weight!

Eat Yourself
SLENDER

NO MORE
- DEPRIVATION
- COUNTING CALORIES
- STARVING YOURSELF
- YO-YO DIETING

My Solution to YOUR Weight Loss Problem: EAT, EAT, EAT !

Barbara A. Hoffman

3. DRINK COFFEE OR TEA:

Caffeine is a central nervous system stimulant, so your daily java jolts can rev your metabolism 5 to 8% That is a nice "bump" Not a coffee fan? A cup of brewed tea can raise your metabolism by 12%. The antioxidant catechins in tea provide the metabolism boost.

4. FIGHT FAT WITH FIBER:

Did you know? Fiber can rev your fat burn by as much as 30%! We all tend to ignore fiber. Instead it should be one of your best friends. Aim for about 25 g a day—the amount in about three servings of vegetables.

5. ALWAYS INCLUDE PROTEIN:

Your body needs protein to maintain lean muscle. Add a serving to every meal and snack. Examples: 3 ounces of lean meat or chicken, 2 tablespoons of nuts, or 8 ounces of low-fat yogurt. Research shows protein can up post meal calorie burn by as much as 35%

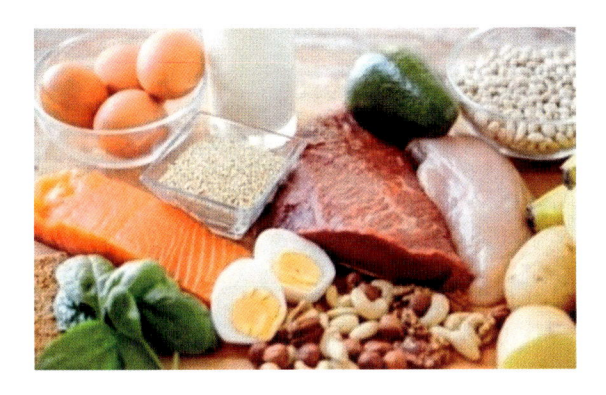

6. GET MORE VITAMIN D:
Did you know? Vitamin D is actually a hormone…it was misnamed many years ago and the "Vitamin" name still prevails. But it is a hormone and hormones are the key messengers of your body! D is essential for preserving metabolism-revving muscle tissue. Unfortunately, researchers estimate that a measly 4% of Americans over age 50 take in enough vitamin D through their diet. You can get 90% of your recommended daily value (400 IU) in a 3.5-ounce serving of salmon. Other good sources: tuna, shrimp, tofu, fortified milk and cereal, and eggs. OR, do what I do…I take 1000-2000 IU of D every day.

2) Shrink Fat Cells

Yes, you can actually shrink fat cells. How? With a substance called Conjugated Linoleic Acid (CLA)

This omega-6 fatty acid has been shown to stimulate fat burn and promote the creation of metabolism-revving lean muscle
There are over 100 studies showing that CLA has a positive effect on those who want to reduce body fat AND maintain lean muscle mass

CLA does this in four distinct ways:
- Decreases the amount of fat that is stored after eating
- Increases the rate of fat breakdown in fat cells
- Increases the rate of fat metabolism
- Decreases the total number of fat cells.

INCREDIBLE benefit… Less fat cells!

CLA also balances blood sugar and curbs the output of hunger hormones to keep cravings at bay. CLA helps to fight and break the yo-yo effect.

Going on vacation and worried about those "Vacation Pounds? Take 1,200 mg of CLA at least once a day throughout your trip.
Researchers found "CLA supplementation among overweight adults significantly reduced body fat over 6 months and prevented weight gain during the holiday season."
Travelers found they came home slimmer than when they left!
An added bonus, CLA has potential anti-cancer properties. Studies have demonstrated that even small amounts of CLA have been shown to slow the growth of a wide variety of tumors, including cancers of the skin, breast, as well as cancers of the lung, prostate, and colon.

I personally take 3 CLA per day for 2 months, then I take a 6 week break and start again for 2 months.

AN IMPORTANT NOTE ABOUT OVER-EATING
Your stomach is about the size of a 6 ounce can. If you enlarge it with a huge meal, it takes **6 weeks of small meals** to return the stomach to normal size! Yikes...now you know what that Thanksgiving dinner can really do! Be Careful!

Chapter 13
Belly Fat and Your Brain

BRAIN BALANCE HELPS DECREASE BELLYFAT

To achieve a flat belly, we need to have hormone balance AND brain balance.

If you work on brain chemistry PLUS your eating habits, you will lose the belly fat.
"Will Power" is not the answer! **"Brain Power"** is the answer. Your brain is "command central" when it comes to weight loss. The brain needs certain nutrients and if it does not get those nutrients, it automatically sends out a hunger signal that results in you OVER-EATING and then your body stores the fat. Where? "The Belly", of course.

The key neurotransmitter balancers are:

- Dopamine
- Serotonin
- GABA

Your Belly Fat / Neurotransmitter Primer

At the end of this chapter, I have a self-test for you

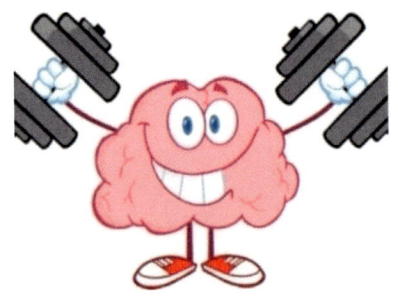

An Overview

> 1. **DOPAMINE – The ENERGY SUPPLEMENT**

LOW DOPAMINE LEVELS = WEIGHT GAIN
Low dopamine symptoms:
• you need more food than a normal person needs to feel "satisfied"
• you often wake up tired
• your energy spikes after eating…so you constantly snack

What happens with low Dopamine?
- Your brain turns to cortisol for energy. When excess cortisol is released, you get puffy and appetite increases. You get bloated and gain weight around the middle because cortisol receptors are located there next to the estrogen receptors.
- Cortisol increases adrenaline…This makes you feel restless, anxious…not able to sleep at night. Lack of sleep prevents your brain from keeping hormones at proper levels and YOU GAIN WEIGHT

- Anxiety causes you to crave comfort foods. You might feel "addicted" to certain food.

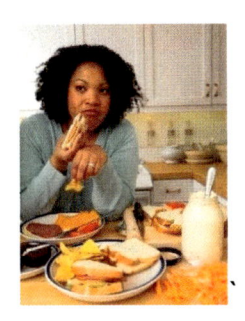

SUGAR DEPLETES DOPAMINE. CUT SUGAR OUT of your diet! To calculate how much sugar is in a particular food, look at the label and find the grams of sugar...Take those grams, divide by the number. The number you get is the number of TEASPOONS OF SUGAR you are ingesting! Wow! This can be shocking & should help you resist high sugar foods.

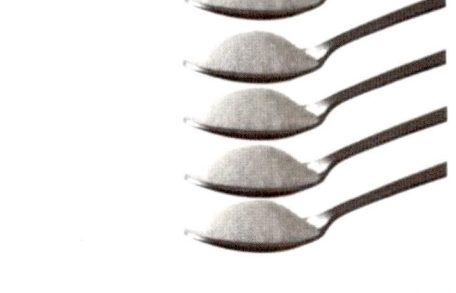

TO INCREASE DOPAMINE NATURALLY
Consume the amino acid tyrosine found in protein-rich meats, poultry, fish, chicken, cottage cheese, eggs, and oat flakes.

Note: a single serving of cottage cheese (½ cup) greatly increases tyrosine which increases dopamine. Try adding some spices. Personally, I like to add chili powder and turmeric.

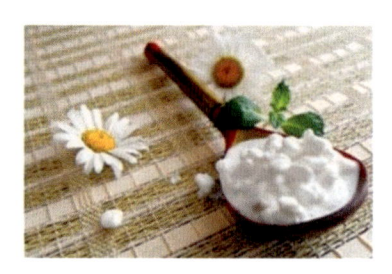

DOPAMINE SUPPLEMENTS:

Phosphatidyl Serine – increases dopamine, lowers cortisol (100-200 mg)
L-Tyrosine – stimulates body to burn up adipose tissue, promotes satiety (500 – 1000 mg)

2. SEROTONIN – The Happiness & Impulse Control Supplement

SEROTONIN MAKES US FEEL SERENE, REFRESHED, HAPPY & HELPS CONTROL CRAVINGS!
When we crave sugar and carbs, we are actually looking for serotonin.

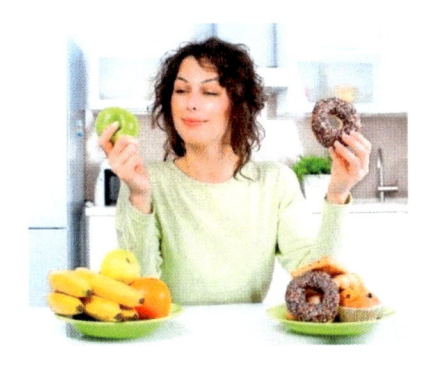

Low Serotonin symptoms:

• You will want carbs with every meal – pasta, potatoes, white breads, rice
• You crave chocolate
• Cravings get worse around time of menstrual cycle
• You consume fewer calories during the day, but at night you raid the refrigerator. You are especially looking for high carb snacks – cakes, crackers, chips, pastries
• You get up and eat in the middle of the night
• You think about food all the time

You are especially vulnerable to:
  • Cravings
  • Panic attacks
  • Sad, depressed mood

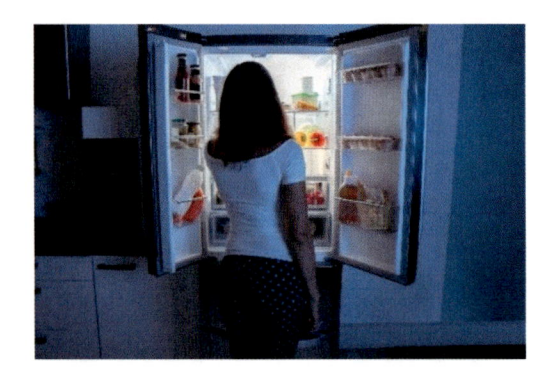

Causes of Low Serotonin:
- Hormone imbalance (low progesterone)
- Environmental toxins
- Stress (eats up serotonin)
- Lack of sleep
- Lack of sun
- Prescription drugs

FOODS THAT INCREASE SEROTONIN LEVELS:
Avocado, chicken, cottage cheese, eggs, yogurt, turkey and wheat germ.

SEROTONIN-ENHANCING HORMONES:
- **Progesterone: 40 – 80 mg per day**
- **Pregnenolone: 50 mg per day**

NUTRITIONAL SUPPLEMENTS TO ENHANCE SEROTONIN:

Melatonin – take at night. It suppresses body weight and visceral fat accumulation the very next day (1.2 – 9 mg)

5-HTP – take at night, reduces appetite, promotes weight loss: 50 – 100 mg

DHEA – Take in the morning, helps burn off belly fat (women: 5 – 20 mg men: 10 – 50 mg)

SAM-e – Take in the morning, can help raise serotonin levels & reduce food cravings: 400 mg

3. GABA – Gamma-Aminobutyric acid– The Brain Calming Supplement

- Promotes Calm, Stable Brain Chemistry
- Keeps you feeling balanced (not tense, irritable, hungry)
- Counteracts emotional eating; stress eating; anxious eating
- Gives control over certain impulses that lead to overeating and bingeing. No more eating in order to control feelings of panic.
- Helps with portion control, over-eating
- Cuts cravings for alcohol/drugs, junk food binges

Low GABA symptoms:

• You have a second helping at every meal
• You binge at a buffet or you can eat a box of cookies in one sitting
• You eat off someone else's plate mindlessly
• You always order dessert just because it is there

GABA ENHANCING HORMONE:
- **Progesterone 40-80 mg per day**

Nutritional Supplements to increase GABA:

GABA is available as a nutritional supplement. Take 550 mg daily. With GABA you can become one of these people you see eating leisurely and laying down their fork without finishing every morsel on their plate. How wonderful! You are under control!

LET'S FIND OUT WHERE YOUR IMBALANCE LIES

Self-Test

Let's pinpoint your needs for success.
Note: You may need more than 1 brain supplement.

IS THIS YOU?

1) I need energy. I am consuming excessive amounts of coffee and sugar to get going and keep going during the day.

You need DOPAMINE
Eat more protein
L-Tyrosine is good for you

2) I binge. I over-eat. I have no portion control. I feel addicted to some foods. When I'm stressed I eat whatever will calm me down. I don't feel like my brain ever tells me to stop eating.

You need GABA
Also, drink green tea (2-4 cups) for calmness, attention, & focus. Decrease caffeine, eat complex carbs & high fiber foods.

3) I often crave salty foods. I am not hungry in the morning, but I can eat all night long. I look for high carb snacks. I get up at night to snack. I eat small snacks, but many of them. I have trouble falling asleep at night.

You need SEROTONIN
5-HTP is especially good for you!
Eat foods high in tryptophan. It is known to increase serotonin very quickly

IN SUMMARY, HERE IS WHAT YOU MAY NEED:

1. Dopamine: **for energy & metabolism**

2. Serotonin: **for a serene, "happy" brain and to eliminate cravings for carbs & salty foods**

3. GABA: **for obsessive/anxious eating patterns & to help you develop portion control**

Chapter 14
Banish Cravings

Cravings contribute to Belly Fat

Banish Cravings! Forever, I promise!

First, let's talk about hunger vs cravings.

Hunger vs Cravings

- When you are **hungry** you want *any* type of food, when you are **craving**, you're craving something *specific*.
- **Hunger-** is the body's way of letting you know it needs fuel; It is a legitimate signal to eat.
- **Cravings-** are generally for a particular food or drink. You might have a craving for chocolate, but not be physically hungry at all. Cravings can be brought on by emotions, unbalanced hormones, unbalanced neurotransmitters, and even memories. You may crave foods to relax, relieve stress or boredom, soothe anger or cope with loneliness
- Hunger:
  - Usually occurs when you haven't eaten for a few hours or more
  - Results in a rumbling stomach, headache or feeling of weakness
  - Doesn't pass with time
  - Isn't just for one specific food

- Cravings:
  - Are usually for comfort foods, such as chocolate, sweets and fatty foods
  - Are often caused by negative feelings
  - Lead to eating that makes you feel good at first, but then guilty
  - May be stronger when you're dieting, especially if you're giving up your favorite foods
  - Can occur even after you've recently eaten

  Cravings will pass with time if you don't "give in"

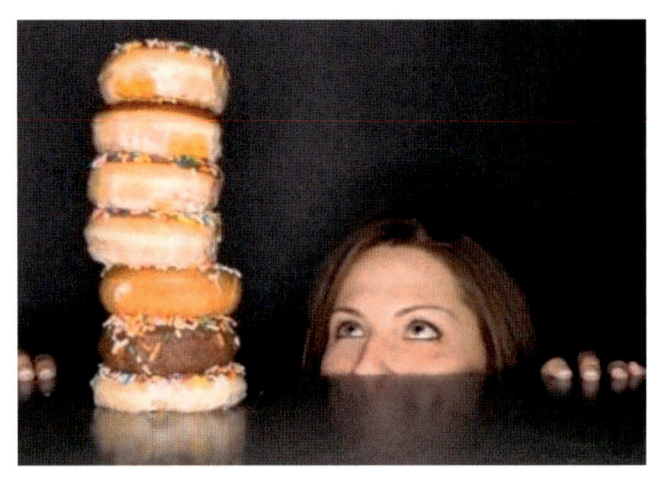

Tips to Give Your Cravings The Cold-Shoulder!
- When a bad craving creeps up on you, take a deep breath, eat 6 walnut halves slowly, OR eat 1 ounce of a good dark chocolate, slowly, savoring the taste.

Also:
- Eating more protein can help lower cravings.
- If you crave carbohydrates like pastas and bread raising your serotonin levels can help minimize the cravings. 5-HTP is your serotonin raising supplement.
- Drinking lots of water and keeping your body hydrated can really help your body brush off the cravings.
- Sleep right! Aim for 7-8 hours per night. You need good sleep for hormones to "reset" properly.

Daily Snack Ideas to Bury Your Cravings!
- Frozen red seedless grapes
- Carrots and hummus
- Apples or any fruit with pectin
- Nuts
- Berries
- Avocado
- Dates with peanut butter
- Nuts
- Green Tea
- A good brand of dark chocolate (some of the best: Dagoba Organic: Eclipse, Whole Foods Dark Chocolate, PMS Chocolate Bars from Art Coco.

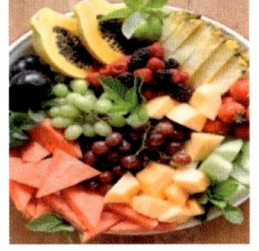

Supplements to Stop Cravings in Their Tracks:

5-HTP
Avena Sativa
L-Tyrosine
Chromemate
PGX

See page 72 for a complete listing of the supplements listed in this book

Chapter 15
Beat the Bloat

BLOATING – Beat the Bloat! Diminish Belly Fat Bloat Quickly

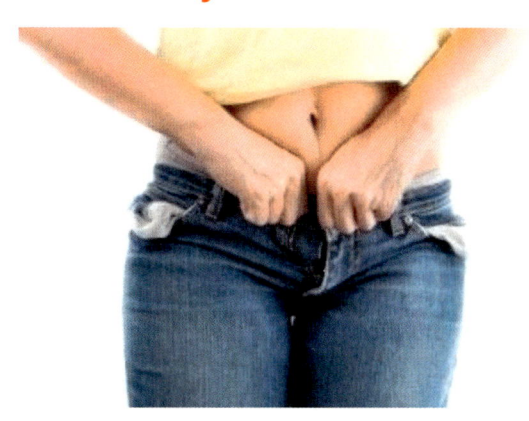

We all have experienced the symptoms of bloating: feeling tight and swollen, sluggish, water-logged, gassy, and of course, the "pants won't fit" scenario.

Here are a few simple ways to combat bloating:
- Progesterone: progesterone is a natural diuretic and reduces / prevents bloating
- Vitamin B6: another natural diuretic which causes excess fluid to be released.
- Increase Protein Intake: Carb-laden foods trigger fluid retention for most of us. Including 3 oz of protein in every meal will help you shed all that unwanted bloat…some people will lose up to 10 pounds when they decrease carbs

and increase protein. Protein slows carb absorption and helps release trapped fluids.
- Greek Yogurt: Greek Yogurt contains more healthy fats and almost twice the amount of protein as regular yogurt. This dynamic duo induces your body tissue to release trapped fluids and reduce bloating by as much as 50%. According to UCLA researchers, a cup of Greek yogurt a day can help shed up to 4 pounds of "false fat" (excess fluid) per week. Greek yogurt also contains digestion-friendly probiotics bacteria which decrease the production of gas, which can cause bloating.
- Iced Tea: Iced tea combines water, caffeine and polyphenols which signal the hypothalamus in the brain to REDUCE the production of vasopressin. Vasopressin is considered the "bloat hormone".

BLOAT-BEATING Belly Flat Veggies and Fruits

To further flatten your belly, load up on these 6 nourishing fruits and veggies:

1. Cucumber
This water-rich veggie will help you minimize any stomach bloat. Cucumbers are "wonder workers" when it comes to reducing puffiness and water retention. Chop up this crispy, refreshing veggie for a snack. Munching on this cool, refreshing, crisp vegetable can eliminate bloating in as little as 3 days. Trapped liquids be gone!

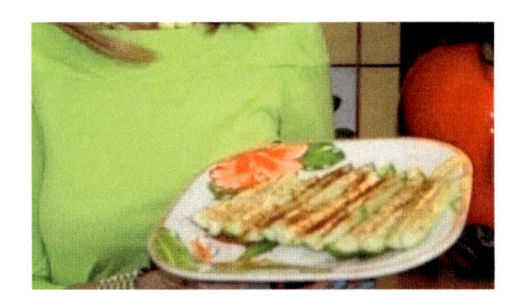

My favorite: sliced cukes sprinkled with Tajin, a glorious Mexican spice

2. Papaya
Papaya contains a bloat-fighting enzyme called papain, which aids in breaking down proteins within the gastrointestinal area, facilitating digestion.

3. Asparagus
This anti-inflammatory and antioxidant-rich veggie is another powerful diuretic that aids in removing extra liquids from the body and helps to reduce unwanted bloat. I lightly steam some spears every week, put them in my fridge and munch on them for a snack.

4. Celery
Celery is another natural diuretic which relieves water retention.

5. Kiwi: The plant acids in kiwi can help shrink your waistline by improving digestion and preventing constipation & gas which are definite belly-swellers.

6. Coconut Water
Coconut water is rich in potassium, a flatulence-fighting mineral and electrolyte that aids in flushing

sodium out of the body. Stick to coconut water that is naturally sweet and doesn't contain any added sugar.

7. Coffee
- Coffee facilitates weight loss because it is a diuretic
- It contains soluble dietary fiber. It loosens bowels and prevents constipation
- Is not unhealthy. Research shows 2-4 cups per day (small cups) is fine
- Enhances metabolism. Helps burn calories & body fat. That is why so many diet products on the market contain caffeine.

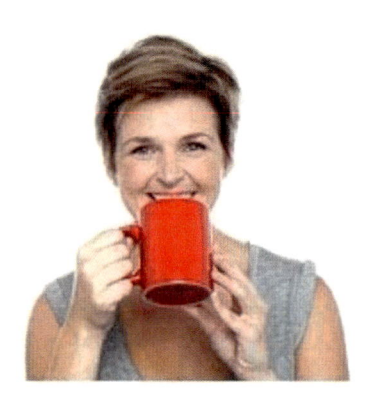

8. Green Tea
- Green Tea contains catechins which stimulate metabolism and fat burning
- You can make your own belly fat burner. Steep 2 green tea bags and 2 black tea bags. Put the tea in a thermos and sip all day.

Chapter 16
Exercise and Belly Fat

WHAT ABOUT EXERCISE?

A NOTE ABOUT EXERCISE.
Do not berate yourself about not exercising at the gym. A significant exercise study followed 3 groups of people:

Group 1 Worked with a trainer for six months
Group 2 Did other miscellaneous exercises like lifting free weights, running, treadmill, etc.
Group 3 Did no particular exercise

Results:
- The trainer group lost only slightly more than the no exercise group
- The miscellaneous exercise group actually gained weight. They noticed they ate more on exercise days!

Another study divided dieters into 2 groups:
Group 1 Dieted only
Group 2 Dieted and exercised 45 minutes 3-5 days/week

The difference was only a couple of pounds!
Diet only group lost 5 – 37 pounds.
Exercise/Diet group lost 8 – 39 pounds.

A compilation of over 43 studies have shown that exercise is not an effective weight loss tool. Of course it IS important to your overall health.

To lose weight the rule of thumb as it stands is EAT LESS, EXERCISE MORE

WHAT YOU SHOULD REALLY DO IS, EAT BETTER & WALK! Walking is great because it gets you into a more healthful mood and it won't make you more hungry!

IS THERE A BELLY FLAT EXERCISE? Yes!

Try this simple "Belly Flat" exercise by Dr. Ellington Darden. It takes less than 60 seconds.

- Lie on your back with hands just below your rib cage.
- Take a normal breath and forcibly Blow all the air out of your lungs for about 7 seconds.
- Then, without inhaling, suck in your ab muscles as hard as you can, as if pulling your navel into your spine.
- Hold for about 10 seconds. This creates a "vacuum effect that powerfully targets a girdle of muscle deep inside your body called the *transverse abdominis*. The tighter this is, the flatter your stomach! Darden recommends using the ab vacuum move twice before each meal.

Once you master the lying position, try it sitting or standing. It will be a bit more challenging, but also more effective. One woman emailed me that she lost 15 inches of abdominal fat in just 12 weeks.

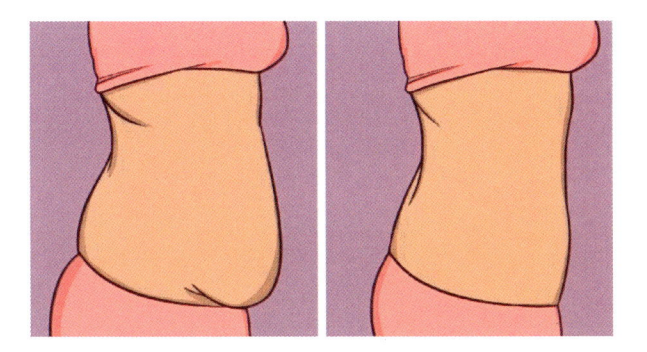

Note:

If you have back pain that prevents you from exercising, you will be pleased to know that when these transverse abdominal muscles are strong, it relieves pressure on the spine that causes back ache.

I use this one, ladies and I LOVE it. You can do it while sitting at your desk or doing your daily chores!

Chapter 17

Estrogen Dominance FAQ's

How do I correct estrogen dominance?

It's not that difficult! Start now, before things get worse!

- The use of natural progesterone crème will usually restore hormonal balance and help a woman "feel like myself" again. Used just 25 days of the month for non-menstruating women and 12 days per month for menstruating women, it can work wonders!
- Avoid external sources of estrogen (xenoestrogens from meats, dairy, plastic, petrochemicals.) Email me for my xenoestrogen handout.

- Use a supplement called DIM (diindolyl methane) or Indole-3-Carbinol which encourages your body to excrete excess estrogens. Good for men, too!

Is there a diet that can help with estrogen dominance?

I have been researching this for some time and have found the following data for you to help eliminate excess estrogens that may be in your body.

- Eliminate conventional dairy foods. Try this for about one month. You might notice a huge difference, especially with breast tenderness. I can tell you from my own experience with fibrocystic breasts that this really works! Spend the extra money for organic milk. It is worth it – especially for your teenagers if they drink a lot of milk.

- Eat cruciferous vegetables in moderate to high amounts broccoli, cabbage, turnips, kale, collard greens, Brussels sprouts. These modulate estrogen levels because they contain indole-3-carbinol.

- Increase fiber: fiber decreases total circulating estrogens! It will pull and hem it right out of the body. You want about 25 grams per day.

- Eat foods high in essential fatty acids (walnut oil, flaxseed oil, sesame oil) or take an EFA supplement

- Meat is okay, but not in copious amounts

- Eat organic vegetables as much as possible. My personal rule: If it something you eat often (for instance, I eat lettuce almost every day), spend the extra money to buy organic.

- Eliminate refined sugar foods. My Sugar Detox is at the end of the book – Chapter

- Low fat foods are best because the higher the dietary fat, the higher the estrogen levels.

Chapter 18
Belly Flat Supplements

RE-CAP OF HELPFUL SUPPLEMENTS
(In alphabetical order)

Avena Sativa - Helps to prevent a sharp increase in blood sugar levels, and improves metabolism to help you feel full. Controls cravings.

Chromemate - helps to regulate blood glucose levels, which prevents carbohydrate cravings.

CLA - Helps reduce body fat mass by decreasing the amount of fat that is stored after eating. It decreases the total number of fat cells, and even increases the rate of fat metabolism.

DHEA - Enhances the thermogenic process of food being transferred into energy instead of fat. DHEA helps you regain muscle mass which increases fat burning.

DIM - Guides used estrogen down the healthy 2-hydroxy pathway. This promotes proper estrogen metabolism in men and women. DIM increases the body's natural ability to burn fat!

GABA - Counteracts emotional and stress eating and gives control over impulses that lead to overeating. Helps with managing portion control.

Magnesium - Triples your odds of keeping weight off permanently. Magnesium spurs the release of fatty acids that you have stored in your midsection. They will now be burned for energy. Magnesium also cuts your stress eating by as much as 50%.

Melatonin - Lowers cortisol. Overly high cortisol in the morning fuels appetite and cravings ALL DAY LONG! When you go into deep sleep, hormones are reset and released. How? Melatonin is released, triggering your body to cool down. When the body temperature drops, the hormones are released and begin to help us regenerate.

L-Tyrosine - Stimulates your body to burn up adipose tissue, promotes satiety, and increases dopamine.

PGX - helps promote healthy blood sugar levels already within the normal range, supports healthy appetite control, and curbs food cravings that are so often to blame for over-indulging and weight gain.

Phosphatidylserine - Works to control cortisol levels and eliminates many of the negative effects associated with elevated levels. Elevated cortisol leads to body fat, and increases appetite and cravings.

Rhodiola Rosea - An adaptogen that helps the adrenal glands produce cortisol in normal patterns, and also increases dopamine.

SAM-e - Increases serotonin levels to cut cravings.

Vitex (Chasteberry) - Directly affects hormone production. Chasteberry stimulates the production of progesterone, which can help to balance hormones. By balancing hormone levels, you can improve appetite and increase energy, all of which make it easier to stick to your Belly Flat regimen.

5-HTP - Increases serotonin levels, which helps to reduce cravings and increase satiety.

If you'd like to take a look at the brands that I've researched, I invite you to visit my website: www.bhnformulas.com

Chapter 19
6 Part Sugar Detox

HOW TO GET OFF SUGAR, PERMANENTLY

Part 1:
THE DETOX OVERVIEW

Okay, let's all lay our cards on the table. Are YOU addicted to Sugar? Do you suspect that you are? Working together, we can BREAK that addiction. I promise you! We will do it in a series of steps that will NOT be painful.

- Do you crave something sweet after every meal?
- Do you crave sweets in the middle of the afternoon?
- Do you have to have sugar in your coffee, tea more than you know you should?
- Do you start your day with something sweet like cereal, pastry or a muffin?

If so, you just might be addicted to sugar ALONG WITH MILLIONS OF OTHER PEOPLE! Sugar addiction can be just as powerful as addiction to drugs like heroin or cocaine. Once the body starts craving it, the cravings demand to be fed. The result of sugar addiction is obesity, specifically Belly Fat, diabetes, heart disease, cancer, loss of brain function, hormone imbalance, PCOS, insulin resistance, premature aging, depression, and anxiety.

SUGAR IS MORE A DRUG THAN A FOOD!

That is why you have to detox from it! Researchers have discovered that sugar and its substitutes can even surpass the reward feeling associated with cocaine use!

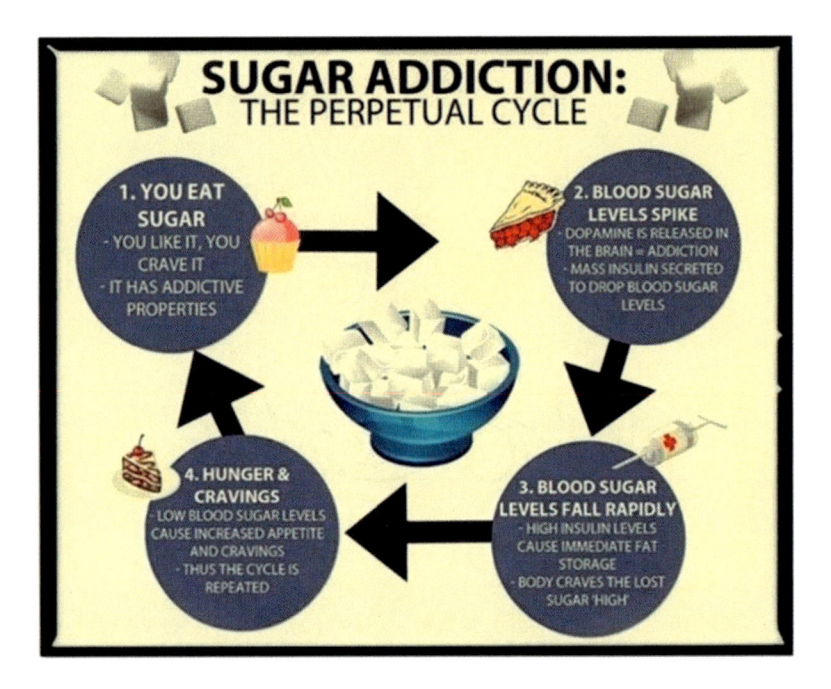

SUGAR ADDICTION: THE PERPETUAL CYCLE

1. **YOU EAT SUGAR**
   - YOU LIKE IT, YOU CRAVE IT
   - IT HAS ADDICTIVE PROPERTIES

2. **BLOOD SUGAR LEVELS SPIKE**
   - DOPAMINE IS RELEASED IN THE BRAIN = ADDICTION
   - MASS INSULIN SECRETED TO DROP BLOOD SUGAR LEVELS

3. **BLOOD SUGAR LEVELS FALL RAPIDLY**
   - HIGH INSULIN LEVELS CAUSE IMMEDIATE FAT STORAGE
   - BODY CRAVES THE LOST SUGAR 'HIGH'

4. **HUNGER & CRAVINGS**
   - LOW BLOOD SUGAR LEVELS CAUSE INCREASED APPETITE AND CRAVINGS
   - THUS THE CYCLE IS REPEATED

HOW DO I KNOW IF I AM ADDICTED?

- I feel moody if I don't eat sugar
- The smell or sight of sugary foods gives me a high or a "rushy" feeling and I begin craving the food
- When I am not eating sugar, I am thinking about it
- I cannot go one day without sugar

- When I do eat sugary foods, I have no impulse control or portion control and I will eat too much
- I experience withdrawal when I go too long without something sugary. This includes headaches, mood swings, irritability, fatigue and feeling depressed

DID YOU KNOW?

- Sugar Addiction is a sign of a brain neurotransmitter deficiency of serotonin and/or dopamine. They are responsible for our search for rewarding foods.
- Neurotransmitter imbalances can be passed down to the 4th generation! So you are not just stopping your own addiction but possibly those of your children and grandchildren. Have you noticed each generation seems to be getting worse with their eating habits? Stop the cycle!

WHAT WILL I DO ON THIS PLAN?

You will slowly decrease the amount of sugar you are using. We will take it one step at a time.

- We will balance your brain's chemistry to beat the feelings of sugar withdrawal. You can notice the difference in as little as 1 week! Over time, you will beat the addiction entirely.

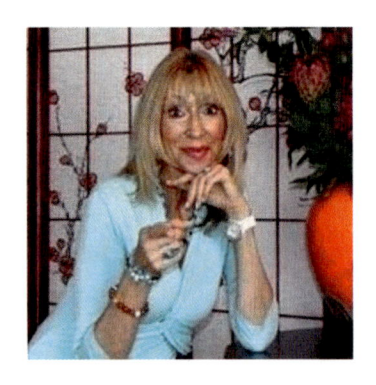

"I did it and I want to help you. It feels fantastic!"
Hugs, Barbara
WHY YOU HAVE SUGAR CRAVINGS:
If you crave sugar, there is a problem with your brain chemistry: your serotonin levels are probably low and the brain is looking to raise them. People will describe the cravings as actually hearing a "white noise" in their head that actually gets louder and louder until they submit to the craving.

GUESS WHAT? That noise can be silenced FOREVER! Nourishing your brain's neurotransmitters with the correct nutrients and balancing your hormones can completely do the trick!

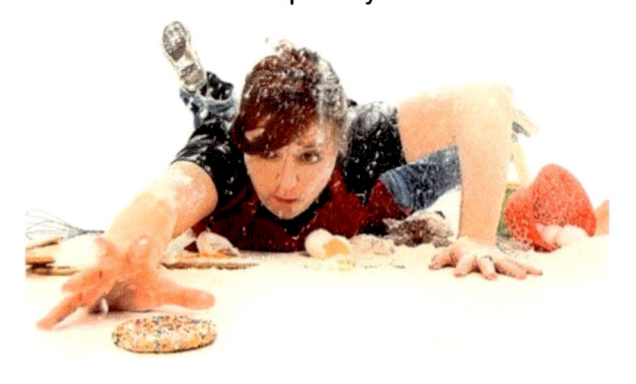

How to start?

Begin reading labels today! Take the grams of sugar for each serving and divide by 4. That equals one teaspoon of sugar! If a carton of yogurt contains 12 grams of sugar, that is 3 teaspoons of sugar! Imagine sitting and eating 3 teaspoons of white sugar for your breakfast or lunch or snack. No wonder people are feeling tired, anxious, depressed or just plain awful! WATCH THOSE LABELS! You can do it easily. Make a game out of it and just REFUSE to purchase those foods or to eat them. Your body is precious and your health is your wealth. Do NOT give it up to sugar!

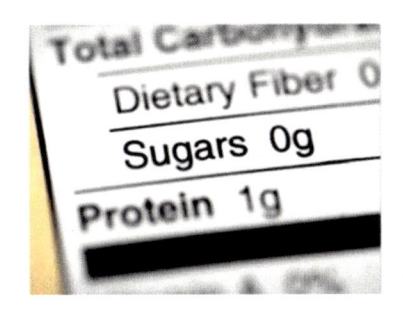

PART 2:

SUGAR BUSTING STEPS AND RULES

Before You Begin Your Sugar Challenge: Some **STEPS** to Take

- Find a buddy to support you
- Tell your friends and relatives what you are doing and ask them NOT to tempt you with sweets
- Have children? Ask them to help you police the foods at the super market. This is how I turned

my son into a proverbial Sugar Cop! If I tried to sneak a sugary substance into my grocery cart, he would take it out…and say "Mom, no!"
- Ask a family member to go on the program with you
- Remember that you are making a WONDERFUL, POSITIVE change in your life. You are Detoxing from a DRUG and you will feel great!
- Remember that you are in control! NOT the sugar!
- If you like to write, keep a journal. Your story can be valuable to help someone else. You could even self-publish it!

TAKE THE SUGAR CHALLENGE: 2 weeks off!

Here are the **RULES** for the 2 week challenge. Follow as many of them as you can! There is no failing! Any elimination of sugar is a good thing.

Try to eat little or no sugar for 6 days, and then give yourself a "Reward Day" on the weekend. After 6 days off sugar, you will begin to notice how SWEET sugar really is!

Do not worry about calories during these 14 days. You are ONLY going to watch your sugar and BREAK THE SUGAR ADDICTION!

NO SUGAR

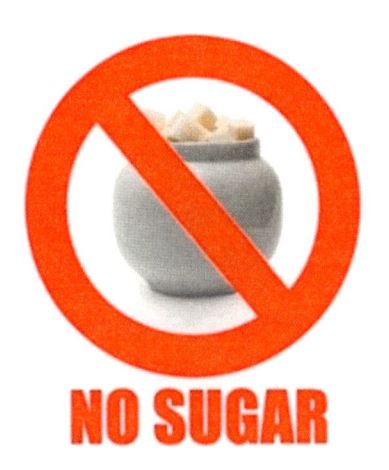

The Easy To Follow Rules

1. Read all labels. Do not eat any food or serving of food that has over 9 grams of sugar. Become a food detective. To reduce sugar, you have to know where it is lurking!
2. Cut the amount of sugar you add to your coffee or tea in half. No artificial sweeteners. They increase cravings. Use real sugar instead if you must.
3. Drink sugar-free herbal teas.
4. Eliminate white rice, white bread, white pasta, which are converted to sugar in the body.
5. Mix any sweet food with a non-sweet food. For instance mix granola with an unsweetened cereal or add extra nuts
6. Do not buy "Fat-free" foods. These are usually loaded with sugar
7. Cut down on salt. Salty foods lead to cravings for sweets

8. Substitute Raisin Bread or Ezekial Bread for breakfast if you are used to a Danish, scone or muffin
9. Eliminate jam or jelly. Fruit spreads still have a lot of sugar. Read the label. Low sugar is okay.
10. Keep nuts, cheese, popcorn, whole grain crackers around for snacks. Be careful of trail mix which can contain sugary components.
11. Try an unsweetened nut butter from the store. Check the sugar grams in peanut butter and be careful!
12. Give up ham and bacon for breakfast because they contain sugar.
13. Eat sliced peaches, strawberries, blueberries as your treat. They may seem expensive, but eat them slowly and savor them. You deserve it!
14. Watch your milk intake because milk contains sugar. Read the label! Rice milk and soy milk are sugary also. Check the label.
15. Stay away from fruit juice. Even the "Unsweetened" ones contain lots of sugar.
16. No commercial salad dressings for these 2 weeks. I bring my own to the restaurant in a little glass bottle. If you have some in your fridge, thin them out with some oil or vinegar.
17. No ketchup because it is LOADED with sugar. Thin it out with some salsa or some sour crème.
18. Eat carrots & hummus. There are some wonderful flavors of hummus. You are crunching & dipping and you will NOT hurt yourself sugar-wise or calorie-wise
19. Do not eat dry-roasted nuts they contain sugar. Eat raw nuts instead.

20. No soft drinks. Choose iced-tea!
21. Be careful with alcohol. It acts like a pure sugar in the body. Dilute it.
22. No syrup-sweetened fruit. If you have some, strain it and rinse it.
23. Freeze some grapes and have those as a snack or eat frozen blueberries
24. No bagels. The flour converts to sugar in the body.
25. Find some good canned soups that are hearty and rich. Check label for sugar
26. Eat turkey and Swiss cheese rolled up with some mustard as a snack. There are countless varieties of mustard and they do not contain sugar.
27. Increase protein. Craving sugar is indicative of not getting adequate protein
28. Microwave a baked potato for a snack. Top with sour cream, salsa, butter, guacamole, or olive oil. This is a great bedtime snack because it helps raise serotonin levels
29. If you are cravings sweets, cook a yam. Great for raising serotonin levels.
30. Do not overdo it with fruit for these two weeks. 1-2 cups per day is the maximum.
31. Reward yourself with chocolate at the end of the day. Make sure it is at least 73% cacao.

Sweeteners; the Good, the Bad, the Ugly

Sugar Has Many Forms: Yup! These can all be bad!

- Agave syrup
- Barley malt

- Maple syrup
- Brown sugar
- Powdered sugar
- Cane sugar
- Raw sugar
- Granulated sugar
- Cane syrup
- High Fructose Corn Syrup
- Rice syrup
- Confectioners sugar
- Honey
- Sugarcane syrup
- Table sugar
- Date sugar
- Turbinado sugar
- Liquid cane sugar
- Sucrose
- Corn Syrup
- Maltose
- Aspartame
- Sweet'N Low
- Splenda

Notes:

1.) Splenda is found in over 4,000 foods & beverages on the market.

Splenda is a chemical! Yes, chlorine is forced into an unnatural bond with a sugar molecule substituting sucrose atoms with chlorine atoms. Splenda begins as a sugar and ends up as a synthetic chemical! Also, it can act as an estrogen mimic in the body. Watch for it and AVOID it please.

2.) Honey is a natural sweetener but has more calories and is actually sweeter than sugar and raises the blood sugar even more than white sugar. Although it does have some medicinal benefits and contains small amounts of minerals, be careful during this phase of your detox.

3.) Agave syrup or nectar is made from the fruit of the agave, a cactus-like plant native to Mexico. It is roughly 75 percent sweeter than sugar. Again, be careful.

Best Sources of Sweetener:

Date "sugar": Made from pulverized dried dates. It is not refined like sugar. It also contains fiber and is high in many minerals. Because the "sugar" is just dried fruit, it is even allowed on sugar-restricted diets for diabetics.

Stevia: has thirty times the sweetness of sugar but it does not raise blood sugar like other caloric sweeteners, so you can use it in moderation.

Sweet Perfection: This is a new sweetener that can be used like sugar in tea, coffee, and baking. It is chicory root ground to a powder that is very high in soluble fiber and looks and tastes exactly like sugar. It will not cause insulin surges.

Are you ready to take the sugar challenge?

Let's go!

1. BE EXCITED FOR YOURSELF! You are embarking on a new adventure. You are taking your body on VACATION! Sugar is an unhealthy, destructive, addictive habit that will rob years from your life.
2. Make yourself a slogan. Mine was "I simply don't eat sugar" I actually was in one of those large warehouse type stores where they give samples. A woman was literally chasing me with a sample of peanut M&Ms on a tray. I simply said "I don't eat sugar" and it REALLY helped me not to even try one and she left me immediately. Yours could simply be "I'm cutting down on my sugar". Whatever sounds reasonable to you.
3. Congratulate yourself at the end of each day. Ask someone else to congratulate you, too.
4. Pick a Bible verse or an inspirational verse that makes you feel good (and STRONG!)
5. Remind yourself. I am going to be less fat and have more energy and I am attacking my Belly Fat.

PART 3:

THE SUGAR-FAT-SALT CONSPIRACY

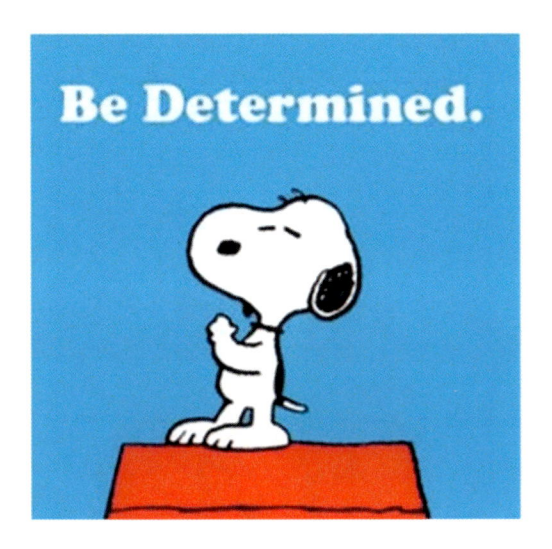

Be Determined.

The "nitty-gritty" of the sugar addiction is the combo of Sugar-Fat-Salt This is EXTREMELY ADDICTIVE.

Combining Sugar/Fat/Salt purposely increases the hedonic value of food (gives immediate pleasure). The sweeter the food, the fattier the food, the more your neurons are stimulated. This prompts a strong emotional response. Your body begins to desire reaching its "Bliss Point" and wants MORE, MORE, And MORE.

The fast food industry knows the addictive properties of sugar and incorporates it into their foods. An example is a crispy food with a salty and sweet taste (chicken nuggets) or a fatty food with a sweet taste (milk shakes). Chicken nuggets are loaded with sugar and fat. Also, did you know that even the hamburger buns have sugar in them? Yes! Also, beef patties can have sugar added as a flavor enhancer.

Fast food french fries: just potatoes right? No! Fast food French fries are frequently dipped in a sugar-solution before frying. Also, the potato breaks down to sugar in your body. When you add ketchup, you add even more sugar.

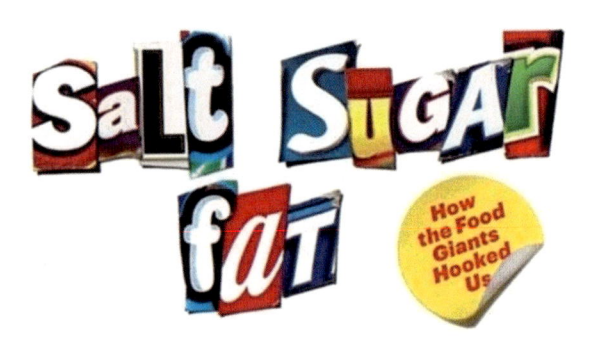

Studies show that laboratory animals will gorge themselves on high fat, high sugar foods, even enduring heavy electrical shocks to get to the sugar. The addiction can get to the point whereby you can drive past a specific location and begin salivating for a specific food that you remember eating. Your body/brain begin incessantly nudging you to stop and GET THAT FOOD. Even a billboard can stimulate some people into impulsive behavior. You become anxious, preoccupied and have to satisfy the urge. Coffee shops have also gotten into the act. Do you crave a regular cup of coffee? Sometimes, but it is 90% of the time the Frappuccino that you crave. This is S-S-F loaded into Coffee! Sugary flavors are manipulated to keep you wanting more and coming back.

PART 4:
SUGAR'S EFFECT ON YOUR BODY

The Effect on Weight
In 1960 the <u>average</u> 40 year old woman weighed 142 pounds.
In 2000 she weighs 169 pounds.
This is frightening! Sugar has changed our entire eating patterns.

With Your Sugar Detox, you can BREAK THE CYCLE.

Sugar & Hormones
Sugar negatively affects the glands which make our hormones. All hormones communicate with each other. When a particular hormone system breaks down, it affects all the other processes in the entire physiological system. Sugar increases insulin levels and increased insulin levels disrupt every other hormone system in the body.

How? When insulin levels are high, too much sugar floods your system. Then you make more insulin. This drives down blood sugar, then you crave sugar. In fact, your body will cry out for sugar. This is a blatant example of the definition of a "viscous cycle".

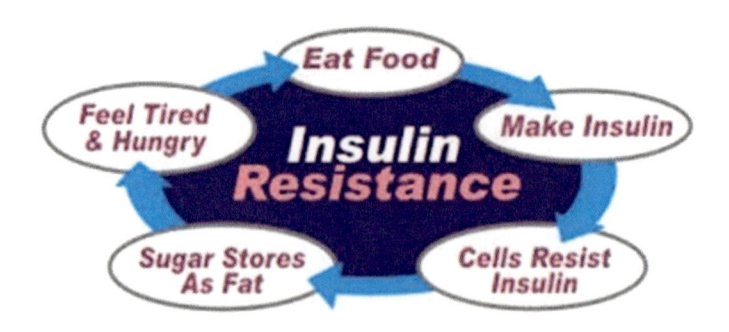

Also increased insulin leads to increased adrenaline and cortisol levels, which means that you now have important hormone levels increased out of their normal ranges.

Sugar & Infertility
If your body is stressed, by a high sugar diet, your sex hormones will become imbalanced, causing your reproductive system to shut down. Stress indicates that it is not a good time to bring offspring into the world because you might not be around to breastfeed and take care of your child. Thus your body interferes with the ability to conceive. Many women stop ovulating when their bodies are not nourished correctly. If you are having infertility problems, CUT OUT THE SUGAR!

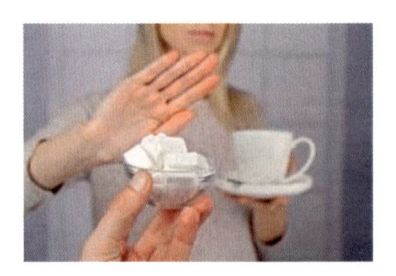

The Lesson: Stay Off Sugar to Keep Your Hormones Balanced!

Now, let us talk about some more medical facts. Knowledge is power!

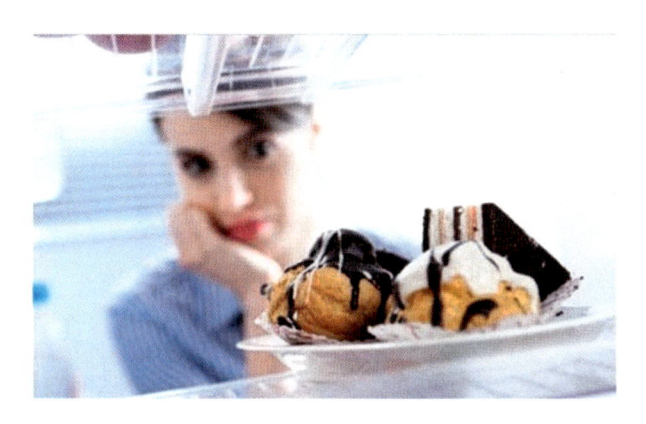

Sugar & Libido
The News is not good! Sugar is a libido-quencher. Sugar-eating people have reported that when they gave in to their sugar cravings, their sex drive "drove off". They have already received a neuro-chemical high from the sweets that they would otherwise have received from sex. Their desire has been fulfilled and the sugar has now taken precedence over their mate. How sad! Don't deplete your libido. STAY OFF SUGAR!

Sugar & Weight
We have countless testimonials from women who have lost weight and dress sizes as well as men who have lost impressive amounts of weight. One lady called last week to say she lost 12 pounds in one month when she gave up sugar and I have told you about my husband who lost 35 pounds in 5 months,

just by eliminating sugars! I myself lost more weight when he went on the program because I became even more vigilant with labels. I did not need to lose weight, but I felt better than ever! A large study showed that eliminating sugar, refined carbs, and also alcohol, for three months, lead to weight loss of up to 100 lbs. seriously! On the other hand, study participants who stepped up their intake of soft drinks and drank one or more per day over the eight years of the study gained, on average, more than 17 pounds. Just by drinking an extra soft drink. Now do you see why American children are overweight? Again, let's break the cycle.

Sugar & PMS
The Connection between Cravings and Carbs. 74 percent of women have cravings when they are pre-menstrual. Nearly 80 percent of the women surveyed wanted high sugar foods. Why? During this time the body's pain threshold is reduced so women are predisposed biologically to crave foods that trigger the release of opioids (morphine like substances) that helps them endure cramps and irritability.

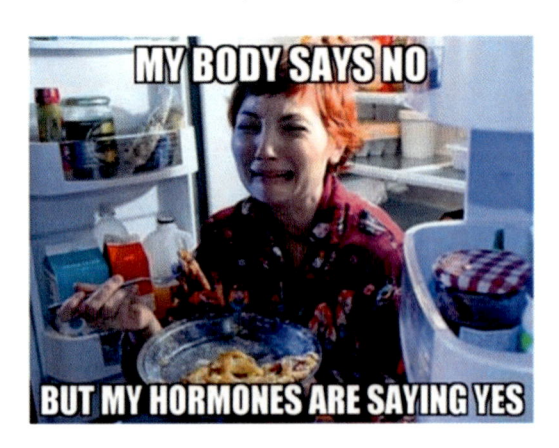

However, the sugar makes them more edgy or depressed. There are hormones and supplements that can do a much better job like natural progesterone and supplements like B-12 and magnesium. Secondly, when we are premenstrual, our serotonin levels drop. Women who feel depressed premenstrually will tend to overeat sweets and other carbs to raise serotonin levels. In other words, we are trying to self-medicate with sugar and carbs. It does not work! It makes you feel worse when your blood sugar subsequently plummets.

A supplement called 5-HTP can naturally raise serotonin levels.

The correct types of carbohydrates, such as yams, can boost serotonin and reduce PMS symptoms. Ladies, managing your sugar intake could be one of the most powerful and effective ways to curtail PMS triggered symptoms.

Sugar & PCOS (Polycystic Ovary Syndrome)
Extra insulin can overwhelm a woman's ovaries to the point where she stops producing progesterone. Instead of progesterone, the ovaries begin to turn out excessive amounts of androgens or "masculine hormones." Androgens and insulin block the development and monthly release of an egg resulting in polycystic ovary syndrome (PCOS), affecting about 10% of women of childbearing age and this is a leading cause of infertility. These androgens cause symptoms such as excess body and facial hair, hair loss, and weight gain. Also, acne and darkening of the skin. With PCOS, a woman may not ovulate for

months at a time and then have a very heavy period. When you create an insulin imbalance your reproductive system can shut down completely.

Committing to a diet of no sugar or quickie carbs is one of the most important changes for a woman with PCOS. Excess insulin causes the body to turn sugar into fat so about 80 to 90 % of women with PCOS are overweight. Excess sugar creates high insulin levels, which stimulate androgen production in the ovary, which suppresses ovulation. The higher LH and the higher androgen levels set up a signal that inhibits the follicle from ovulating. Because each follicle grows and creates a lake of fluid around it, if it does not burst and release its egg, a cyst is left. Therefore you get into a situation of high or normal estrogen levels, high androgens, and low progesterone. Again, PCOS is usually characterized by obesity, especially middle-of-the-body obesity, androgen signs such as acne, oily skin, facial and breast hair and head hair loss. Avoid sugar and refined carbs!

Sugar & Wrinkles: Low Sugar = Fewer Wrinkles
Sugar is very damaging to the skin because sugar molecules attach to collagen fibers, causing them to become stiff and inflexible. This leads to wrinkling, a leathery look, and loss of elasticity of your skin. Glycogen also discolors skin so dark patches may appear. Our bodies are quite miraculous: Collagen can be rebuilt. Stop eating sugar and the free radicals will reduce, and the damage to collagen will reduce. If you took some skin cells, put them into a Petri dish, and let them grow, and then added a few drops of sugar, inflammatory chemicals go up by 1,000 percent over the baseline of one hour. Scientists also

link other skin conditions to excessive sugar and processed carbs. Skin tags those little flaps of skin that crop up in the armpit, neck, or groin area are "external symptoms of insulin resistance."

Sugar & Hair Loss
Too many sugary foods and refined carbs coupled with stress increase the levels of cortisol and testosterone. This causes hair loss as well as dull-looking hair. The hair loss is diffuse and excessive - from the entire scalp. If you are eating too much sugar, metabolic processes slow down. High sugar, low-fat diets lead to low-thyroid activity which translates to hair loss. GIVE UP SUGAR FOR THICKER, HEALTHIER HAIR!

Sugar & Adrenal Fatigue
If you are a sugar addict, your life is always in crisis. When you feel burned out by stress or the demands of life, you reach for sugar. Your adrenal glands are tired, but you use sugar to bolster your energy. This will backfire because you are driving your adrenals even harder.

Finally, your cortisol levels are exhausted and your immune system lies down on the job. Sugar cravings increase.

Did you get the medical message? I hope so. Avoid sugar to the best of your ability and you are on your way to Better Health…I promise you.

Part 5:
HIDDEN SUGAR – IT'S EVERYWHERE

Let's take a look and see if you have too much sugar lurking in your house!

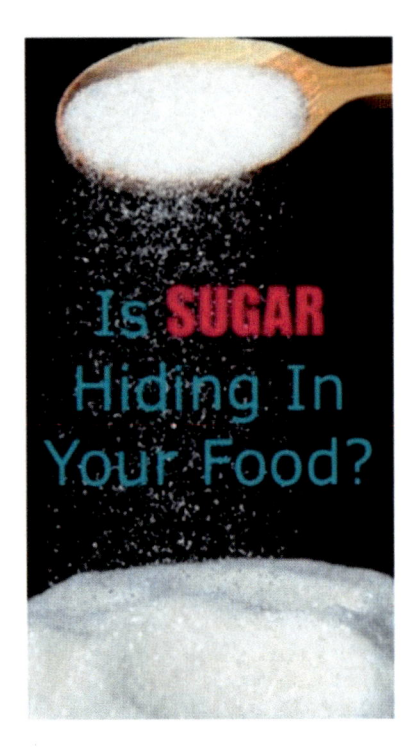

Avoid these HIGH SUGAR FOODS
(Some you will recognize, some will surprise you!)

- Flavored popcorn
- Cocoa
- Fruit butters
- Fruit leathers
- Jello - this is pure sugar!
- Granola bars or granola

- Energy bars - some are just "dressed up" candy! Also, many contain chemicals. Some are low sugar. Look for those.
- Honey
- Ice cream
- Jams, jellies, marmalade
- Molasses
- Processed yogurt, flavored yogurt. Choose Greek Yogurt
- Sherbet
- Syrups
- Fruit juice: 12 ounces of some have the same amount of sugar as a 12 oz soda
- Gatorade (has 14 grams of sugar in 8 ounces)
- Ensure
- Soy milk, rice milk. Almond milk is best choice but still has sugar.
- Carnation Instant Breakfast- 22 grams per serving!
- Bacon
- Muffins
- Flavored vinegars
- Alcohol
- Tonic water - LOTS of sugar in it!
- Syrup sweetened fruit
- Anything "fat free"
- Croissants, white toast, some bagels
- BBQ sauce
- Hoisin sauce / oyster sauce
- Ketchup
- Relishes
- Sweet pickles
- Gravies

You want to AVOID the following fats that contain BOTH sugar and chemicals:

- Bottled salad dressings
- Imitation mayonnaise or sour cream
- Margarine
- Non-dairy creamers
- Pressurized whipped cream
- Cream substitutes, flavored and unflavored

Glycemic Index
Some of you have asked me about this and it does have popularity among some medical doctors and authors of diet books. It actually comes down to common sense when choosing your foods, but here is how the GI works.

The GI is a numerical system of measuring how quickly a food triggers a rise in blood glucose. The score of pure glucose = 100. All other foods are measured in relation to this.
In other words, WHAT IS THE SUGAR CONTENT OF THIS FOOD? The Glycemic Index will tell you.
The higher the GI number, the more the glucose is released in a surge which triggers dramatic spikes in blood sugar. The lower the GI, the more gradual the-release of the glucose. LOWER GI IS BETTER! If you want to use the GI index as a tool, gravitate toward foods with lower numbers and you will be on the road to STAYING OFF SUGAR!

You want to stay away from foods with a GI of 70 or higher because they provide the heftiest surge in blood sugar. Choose foods with a GI of 55 or less because they trigger a small, steady rise in blood sugar. These are most vegetables, legumes, whole grains, and low-sugar foods. You can judiciously select foods with a GI between 56-69, which cause a slightly higher glycemic response. These can be your TREATS.

Sometimes some good vitamin-rich foods have a higher glycemic index than might be considered advisable. These include pineapples, bananas, mangoes, papayas, cantaloupes, and watermelons. Balance these foods and you can still eat them. If a fruit contains a higher glycemic index than sugar-rich ice cream, which would you choose? The unrefined fruit, of course!

You choose to use the GI if you wish. There are many charts available in books and on the Internet, but you do not need the GI if you are choosing high-quality carbs. Reduce white flour foods as best you can. If you simply must eat a "white" food, choose those that give you the least pleasure so no addiction is triggered.

Classification	GI range	Examples
High GI	70 and above	Baked Potatoes, White Bread, Rice Pasta, Corn Flakes, Fruit Roll-Ups, Sports Drinks, Bagels, Rice Cakes, Dates, Soda Crackers, Doughnut
Medium GI	56–69	Macaroni & Cheese, Table Sugar, Brown Rice, Sweet Potato, Banana, Raisins, Grapefruit Juice Unsweetened
Low GI	55 or less	Most Fruits and Vegetables, Beans, Whole Grains, Meat, Eggs, Milk, Nuts, Fructose and Products Low in Carbohydrates

Suggestion:
For the first 3 weeks, avoid high glycemic fruits and veggies: corn, raisins, bananas, grapes, watermelon, potatoes, beets, and mango. Then you can introduce them in small portions. Watch how you feel. Also watch for weight gain, if that is an issue for you.

What happens when we cut out sugar?

At first you may feel moody or irritable. This will pass in 7-10 days and you can ease yourself thru this. To navigate your transition, eat THE BEST DARK CHOCOLATE YOU CAN FIND!
Good dark chocolate does not breakdown collagen and elastic tissue like sugary chocolate does. Dark chocolate is great because it has no milk and less sugar. If you are craving a sweet, go for dark chocolate-covered almonds. Those are the best!

PART 6:
8 KEYS TO YOUR SUCCESS

#1 PROTEIN, PROTEIN, PROTEIN! (with some fat)
It is possible to overeat Carbohydrates, but you really cannot overeat Proteins and Good Fats, so don't worry. START YOUR DAY WITH A PROTEIN - every day!

The Good News About Protein:
Protein curbs hunger so you do not overeat and snack too much between meals. Protein takes longer to break down in your body and keeps you satisfied longer. Researchers in France found that high-carb snackers got hungry JUST AS QUICKLY as people

who had NO SNACKS AT ALL. Those who snacked on chicken (protein) stayed full almost 60 minutes longer. Now, that is significant! Protein improves insulin and glucose levels, so it protects you against Insulin Resistance. Protein is mostly burned for energy and NOT stored as fat like carbs.

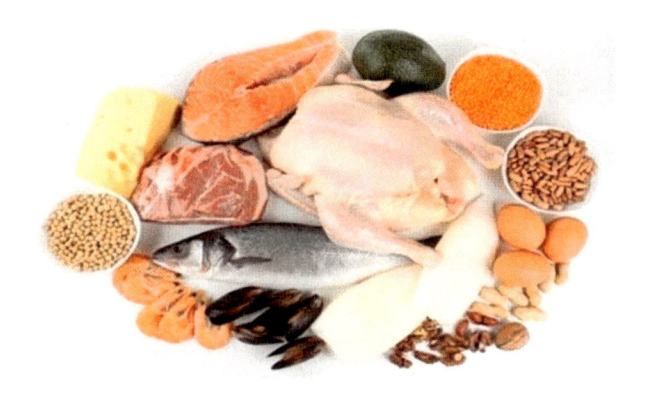

#2 NO LOW FAT DIETING!
When you eat a low-fat diet, your intake of carbs increases, causing high levels of sugar. This excess sugar is converted to triglycerides and is often stored as fat. Years of a low fat diet results in shrinking of muscle mass, less dense bones, increased blood pressure, increased cholesterol and weight gain. You need fats, you do NOT need sugar.

#3 NEVER LET YOURSELF GET TOO HUNGRY.

#4 NO SODAS, NOT EVEN DIET.
Even diet sodas promote sugar cravings.

#5 WHEN YOU HAVE A CRAVING, EAT SOMETHING THAT IS NOT SWEET.
Try eating a sour pickle or something hot. It can trick your brain into losing the craving. I like to cut up cucumbers, put some olive oil and vinegar and some hot chili peppers on them. Hot foods also raise your metabolism.

#6 GET A BUDDY TO GIVE UP SUGAR WITH YOU.

#7 SWEETEN FOODS WITH STEVIA.
Stevia rebaudiana bertoni is the leaf from a shrub in the chrysanthemum family that is grown in South America and Asia. Stevia is about 150 to 300 times sweeter than sugar, has zero calories, and doesn't raise blood sugar levels

#8 JUST PLAIN OLD HUNGRY?
My Number One go-to food is pizza. Yes, that's right! Ask for whole-wheat, thin crust, light cheese (I like extra sauce) and pile on the veggies. This is a good protein low-fat snack without a lot of calories. One piece can be about 200 calories and you will feel FULL!

A note about the children in your life:

I have seen kids, on a limited lunch hour at school, hop into a car, drive 15 miles to a favorite fast food place, grab the food and eat it in the car on the way back without even getting out of the vehicle! Tell your-kids that it is NOT food if it comes in thru the car window!

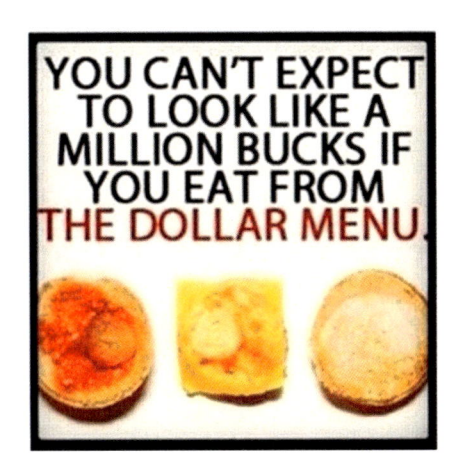

> YOU CAN'T EXPECT TO LOOK LIKE A MILLION BUCKS IF YOU EAT FROM THE DOLLAR MENU.

What can you do for your children / grandchildren / nieces & nephews

- Make a rule: We do not eat in the car.
- Scare your kids. I had my son read Fast Food Nation when he was 14 and he refused to go into a fast food restaurant after that. Truly, there are some disgusting passages in that book. It worked for our family! He was able to resist peer pressure after reading it, which is really hard to do!
- Studies say that we are the first generation whose kids will die younger than we do. Say to yourself, "Not MY kids!"

Supplements

What are the best supplements for sugar control and cravings?
(These also help with weight loss in general)

5-HTP: 50 mg per meal
L-Tyrosine: 500-1000 mg
Zen Mind (GABA): 500-100 mg
Vitamin B-12
Avena Sativa (for cravings)
Fish Oils
Chromium
L-Tyrosine: Raises Dopamine levels (For impulsive eaters/ sluggish metabolism)

My Favorite Success Story: Jack LaLanne

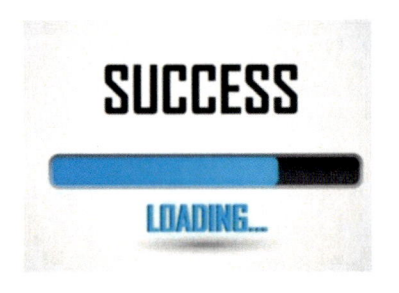

LaLanne's father died of a heart attack at age 50. His mother began to spoil him, giving him sweets as a reward. By the time he reached adolescence he had become a "sugarholic" with a violent temper and suicidal thoughts. But that was only the beginning: He was failing in school, his stomach was upset, he wore glasses, he had terrible headaches, he was weak and skinny and he had pimples and actual boils. "I was demented! I was psychotic! It was like a horror movie!" LaLanne said of this time of his life.

When he was 15, his distressed mother dragged him to a lecture on healthful living being given by nutritionist Paul Bragg. At some point Bragg asked the young LaLanne what he had eaten for breakfast, lunch and dinner, and Jack replied: "Cakes, pies and ice cream!" "He said, 'Jack, you are a walking garbage can." But Bragg offered nutritional salvation to LaLanne: He could be "born again" and be the healthful and strong person he wanted to be - if he changed his ways.

LaLanne took Bragg's message fully to heart. And, by his own testimony and that of everyone around him, he never had cake, pie, ice cream or any sweet from that day forward. All his maladies disappeared; he even stopped wearing glasses. "I was a whole new human being," he said of this transformation. "I liked people, they liked me. It was like an exorcism, kicking the devil outta me!"

Wow! What a testimony.

If you are having any difficulty, I sincerely hope you are reaching out for the support you need. I truly enjoy hearing from you and being your cheerleader as we go forth, so do not hesitate to call me! My husband is now celebrating one year without sugar and he looks and feels like a new man. I am into my 5th year and when I celebrated my birthday this year, I felt like the clock was turning back, not ahead! My mood and energy and weight are completely stable and I feel fantastic! As a former carb/sugar-a-holic, I want this for you!

Chapter 20
Final Thoughts

Barbara, How can you help me personally beyond this book?

Friends, I am available to help you fight the Belly Fat. I have helped many other women and I want to help you. You can call my office and schedule a free phone chat with me. No sales involved, just information and support.

My numbers are 877 880-0170 and 844 539 6200. My wonderful assistants will be happy to work out a time when we can speak.

MOST EFFICIENT: Email me your questions: barbara@askbarbarahoffman.com. I promise to answer within 48 hours. If you are struggling with weight, you might want to email me a food diary for the past 7 days. I can help you pinpoint your weight loss sabateurs. Sometimes there are simple foods that are blocking you.

I also encourage you to check out my book, Eat Your Self Slender on Amazon if you want specific tips for a higher protein, lower carbohydrate diet.

You can do it!

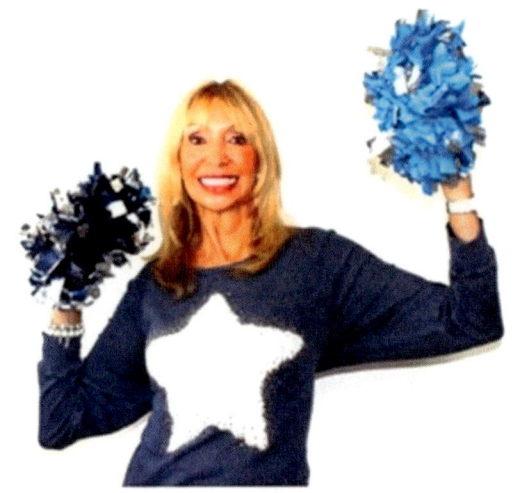

Call or email me if you need help!

barbara@askbarbarahoffman.com

I promise to answer!

877-880-0170

Made in the USA
Columbia, SC
23 June 2019